Plant Based Diet Meal Plan

A Beginner's Guide to Plant Based Nutrition for Weight Loss and for Healthy Mind with Easy and Whole Recipes

Sophia Scott

1

Legal & Disclaimer

The information contained in this book and its contents is not designed to replace or take the place of any form of medical or professional advice; and is not meant to replace the need for independent medical, financial, legal or other professional advice or services, as may be required. The content and information in this book has been provided for educational and entertainment purposes only.

The content and information contained in this book has been compiled from sources deemed reliable, and it is accurate to the best of the Author's knowledge, information and belief. However, the Author cannot guarantee its accuracy and validity and cannot be held liable for any errors and/or omissions. Further, changes are periodically made to this book as and when needed. Where appropriate and/or necessary, you must consult a professional (including but not limited to your doctor, attorney, financial advisor or such other professional advisor) before using any of the suggested remedies, techniques, or information in this book.

Upon using the contents and information contained in this book, you agree to hold harmless the Author from and against any damages, costs, and expenses, including any legal fees potentially resulting from the application of any of the information provided by this book. This disclaimer applies to any loss, damages or injury caused by the use and application, whether directly or indirectly, of any advice or information presented, whether for breach of contract, tort, negligence, personal injury, criminal intent, or under any other cause of action.

2

You agree to accept all risks of using the information presented inside this book.

You agree that by continuing to read this book, where appropriate and/or necessary, you shall consult a professional (including but not limited to your doctor, attorney, or financial advisor or such other advisor as needed) before using any of the suggested remedies, techniques, or information in this book.

Table of Contents

Introduction

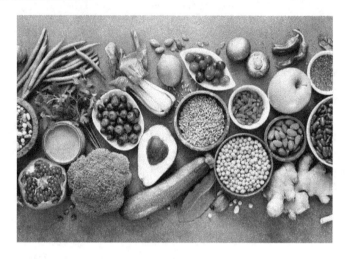

Selecting the perfect diet plan can be confusing thanks to the variety of diet plans available these days. Irrespective of what diet plan you opt for, almost all nutritionists and dietitians across the globe recommend diet plans that limit processed foods and that are based more on whole and fresh foods. The Plant-Based Diet is based on these universally preferred foods.

The primary focus of a plant-based, whole-food diet plan is to minimize the intake of processed foods as much as possible and consume more plant-based, whole natural foods that are proven to be beneficial for not only improving your health but also stimulating effective weight loss. This introduction is going to clear away all ambiguities and doubts regarding the whole-food, plant-based diet plan and provide logical explanations to the benefits it offers.

The whole-food plant-based diet plan is more flexible and understanding than other diets, too. It is mostly comprised of plant-based foods, but you can also have some animal-based products. The extent of animal-based foods in your diet plan depends on your personal choice to entirely not eat them or to consume them in moderation. In general, the more of your plant-based meals, the more beneficial the diet will be for you.

Scientific studies have proven the fact that eating animal products increases the risk of heart disease, cancer, diabetes, obesity, and Alzheimer's disease. The increased risk of suffering from these ailments means that one's lifespan can be considerably reduced. In terms of heart disease, animal products such as dairy products and meat are high in saturated fats. Consuming these products raises cholesterol levels in our bodies. Accordingly, there is a high possibility that arteries could block. The effect of this is that one could likely suffer from a heart attack. What's more, a stroke could occur, as there is limited blood supply to the brain.

Now knowing that eating animal products is a huge risk to your health, it definitely stands as a solid reason why you should opt for plant-based foods. Besides improving your overall health, these foods have numerous benefits to your body. First, they are rich in fiber. Therefore, your digestion will be improved. Their high fiber content, however, demands that dieters should slowly change their usual meals because the bodies take time to adapt.

Plant-based foods are also an ideal choice when one is looking to lose weight. It is disheartening to learn that about 69% of the adult population in the United States is obese. This is a worrying statistic, especially bearing in mind that obesity is linked to cardiovascular diseases and diabetes. Adopting a plant-based diet can help in promoting weight loss. The great thing about this is that you will lose weight naturally without having to worry about gaining again in the future. Usually, the fad diets that people rush to rely on have long-term negative effects. Most people complain about gaining more weight after they had initially shed some pounds. Eating plant foods could prevent such effects.

A diet composed only of plants will be beneficial in maintaining healthy skin. Providing your skin with the nutrients it requires is the best way of keeping it smooth and glowing. Unfortunately, people lack information about this. As such, they are forced to try different skin products with the hopes of giving their skin a natural glow and clear complexion. Eating right is a solution to almost every disease that we might be suffering from. We have been blinded by the media from realizing that the cure we need is in our food choices.

Chapter 1: Plants and Your Health

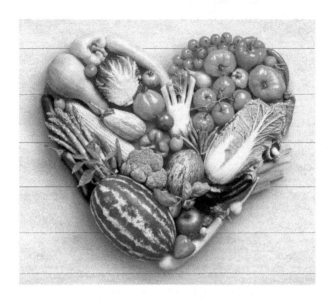

Plants as a Medicine

Medicine has always been made using plants. It is therefore crystal clear that the plant-based diet can serve as medicines to our bodies.

You may find that when a person is unwell, a health expert may recommend eating a particular plant-based food. This is because plants have always had medicinal properties.

Diet-Related Diseases

Some of the diseases that are diet-related include;

- Diabetes

- Cancer

- Cardiac arrest

Foods that Increase Inflammation

Saturated Fats

By now, everyone knows that saturated fats are not good for your body, but the danger is doubled for individuals with chronic inflammation. First, saturated fats easily add weight, one of the primary triggers for inflammation. Secondly, several studies have concluded that a high intake of saturated fats prevents substances in white blood cells from telling them to go dormant. Too much saturated fat keeps the white cells revved up in search-and-destroy mode instead of standing down in recognition that there is no longer any danger present.

Trans Fats

Even more important, avoid trans fats. These are foods labeled as hydrogenated or partially hydrogenated oils. They include vegetable shortening, margarine, crackers, cookies, etc. Vegetable and seed oils may be processed with chemicals and should be avoided. Oils to avoid are soy, corn, sunflower, saffron and palm oils.

Processed foods are also considered "bad" foods because they are frequently filled with chemicals that are "foreign" to your body. This would include protein bars, whipped spreads and even hot dogs. They are also present in pasteurized, dried, smoked, and grilled foods.

Fried foods are usually high in unhealthy fats, making them very bad for individuals with chronic inflammation. Fried foods contain Advanced glycation end products (AGEs). AGEs are created by the high-temperature frying process and are a major contributor to inflammation. Of course, this includes french fries, fried chicken, and fish sticks (sorry).

Grain-Fed Meat

These animals are fattened quickly without the benefit of natural grasses. And, on a humanitarian note, the animals are usually confined to small areas and are seldom allowed out to exercise or see the light of day. Another problem is that these "manufactured" animals are fed antibiotics, which we then consume in the process of eating them for dinner. Those antibiotics can hang out in our bodies and trigger all sorts of inflammation.

Dairy

Many people have allergies to dairy products; if you have a reaction to dairy, you probably are experiencing a form of chronic inflammation. Dairy products can also increase your blood sugar. Higher blood sugar contributes to chronic inflammation. The solution is to limit your intake of cheese, milk, and other dairy products. The exception is unsweetened yogurt, which is on the good food list. Although yogurt is a dairy product, it contains probiotics that help to reduce inflammation.

Sugar

Refined sugar makes the body sluggish and it can wreak havoc on your immune system. When your antibodies come out to fight a problem, they have trouble going away because they just don't care anymore. Excessive glucose in your system slows down your digestive system, which prevents the white blood cells from getting enough energy to kill germs.

Sugar can make you susceptible to infections. You more easily come down with colds, the flu and other bugs. It also makes you more susceptible to cancer. Sugar raises blood sugar levels and contributes to obesity. For these reasons, it is best to avoid anything high in refined sugar content, such as baked goods, soft drinks, and definitely anything with high fructose corn syrup on the ingredients list.

This means you'll want to avoid snack bars, candy, coffee drinks, sweet tea, pies, cakes and all those really good tasting items. This doesn't mean you can't have any. Just cut way back, making them only a tiny percentage of everything you eat.

Starches

Starches can include anything made with flour, especially if it's refined. The refining process for flour strips the grain of valuable nutrients. This "refinement" also makes it harder for your body to digest these foods, by putting them in a form that is harder for your body to convert to fuel. The process can spike blood sugar, which in turn prompts your pancreas to dump large amounts of insulin into your system, taxing both your pancreas and your circulatory system. Starches include white rice, barley, rye, wheat, and products like pretzels, flour tortillas, cereals, and bread.

Vegetables like corn, peas, and potatoes are also considered starches. You have probably heard of people with celiac disease or gluten intolerance. These are just another form of chronic inflammation.

At-A-Glance, here is the "Bad" Food List which increases Inflammation:

- Fried foods including chicken, fish, and french fries

- Any fast food including burgers and wraps

- Egg rolls (fried)

- Hot dogs

- Bacon

- Margarine

- Vegetable shortening

- Red meat

- Pork

- Sausage

- Cold cuts

- Jerky

- Whipped spreads

- Vegetable, soy, corn, sunflower, saffron or palm oil

- Pizza

- Spice mixes

- Bagels

Foods that Reduce Inflammation

If you already eat a fairly healthy diet, you will have no trouble incorporating these foods into your meals. In fact, you may already be enjoying them and just need a few tweaks to increase their presence in your meal planning. Some of the good foods that prevent and reduce chronic inflammation are as follows:

Omega 3 Fatty Acids

Omega 3 fatty acids are found in fish and fish oil. They calm the white blood cells and help them realize there is no danger, so they will return to dormancy.

Fruits And Vegetables

Most fruits and vegetables are anti-inflammatory. They are naturally rich in antioxidants, carotenoids, lycopene, and magnesium. Dark green leafy vegetables and colorful fruits and berries do much to inhibit white blood cell activity.

At least nine servings of fruits and vegetables each day are recommended. One serving is about a half-cup of cooked fruits and vegetables or a full cup if raw. The Mediterranean Diet, rich in fruits and vegetables, is often suggested to individuals suffering from chronic inflammation.

Protective Oils And Fats

Yes, there are a few oils and fats that are actually good for chronic inflammation sufferers. They include coconut oil and extra virgin olive oil.

Fiber

Fiber keeps waste moving through the body. Since the vast majority of our immune cells reside in the intestines, it is important to keep your gut happy. Eat at least 25 grams of fiber every day in the form of fresh vegetables, fruits, and whole grains. If that doesn't provide enough fiber, feel free to take a fiber supplement.

Miscellaneous

Flavor your food with spices and herbs instead of bad fats and unsafe oils. Spices like turmeric, cumin, cloves, ginger, and cinnamon can enhance the calming of white blood cells. Herbs like fennel, rosemary, sage, and thyme also aid in reducing inflammation while adding delicious new flavors to your food.

Healthy snacks would include a limited amount of unsweetened, plain yogurt with fruit mixed in, celery, carrots, pistachios, almonds, walnuts, and other fruits and vegetables.

Plants for Weight Loss

Obesity is considered to be an epidemic nowadays. Shockingly, more than 69 percent of adults in the United States are considered obese or overweight. Making changes in your diet and your whole lifestyle can lead to drastic weight loss when done properly. The impacts of these changes can be promising and long lasting. There are numerous studies that determined plant-based diet plans are very effective for weight loss.

The whole-food plant-based diet plan is rich in fiber and restricts processed foods while forbidding soda, refined grains, fast food, candy, and added sugars, making it ideal for weight loss. An overall assessment of 12 research studies found that people who followed plant-based diet plans lost more weight (2 kg less, in almost 18 weeks as compared to non-plant-based diet followers). Therefore a plant-based diet plan can also keep you from gaining weight.

Chapter 2: Benefits of Plant Based Diet

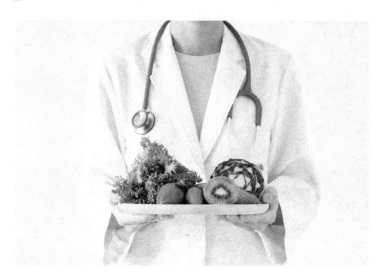

Lowers Blood Pressure

The plant-based diet is known to lower blood pressure. This is due to the fact that the plant-based diet has very little amounts of sugars, which aid in raising the blood pressure. If you have a condition of high blood pressure, a plant-based diet is the right remedy for you.

Lowers Cholesterol Level

Let me start by asking you a question; how much do you think one egg affects your cholesterol? One egg a day could increase your dietary cholesterol from 97 to 418 mg in a single day! There was a study done on seventeen lacto-vegetarian college students. During this study, the students were asked to consume 400kcal in test foods along with one large egg for three weeks. During this time, their dietary cholesterol raised to these numbers. To put it in perspective, 200 to 239 mg/dL is considered borderline high.

The next question you should be asking yourself is what is considered a healthy amount of cholesterol? The answer is zero percent! There is no tolerable intake of trans fats, saturated fats, nor cholesterol. All of these (found in animal products) raise LDL cholesterol. Luckily, a plant-based diet can bring your cholesterol levels down drastically. By doing this, you will be lowering your risk of disease that is typically related to high cholesterol levels. The good news here is that your body makes the cholesterol you need! There is no need to "get it" from other sources.

Did you know that over 69% of the adult population in the United States is obese? This is a worrying statistic as it means that more than half of the adult population is suffering. Additionally, they face the risk of suffering from hypertension and other cardiovascular diseases. Fortunately, there is a remedy for this. Simply changing your lifestyle and your diet can promote weight loss. That's not all; your overall health will also improve.

Plant-based diets have shown that they can aid in considerable weight loss due to their rich fiber content. The absence of processed foods in these diets also provides a huge boost in shedding those pounds.

A plant-only diet will also ensure that you don't gain weight in the long term. Unfortunately, numerous weight loss plans out there only help people in the short term, and individuals end up gaining more weight when they fail to stick to the weight loss plans. Therefore, with regard to sustainability, a plant-only diet is an ideal option.

Maintains Healthy Skin

We all know people who try every skin product imaginable just to get clear, smooth skin. What these people fail to understand is that how we look is more or less dictated by our food choices. Consequently, plant-based diets have a higher chance of providing your skin with the nutrients it needs to stay healthy. For instance, tomatoes provide the body with lycopene. This component safeguards the skin from sun damage. Sweet potatoes are known to provide us with vitamin C. The production of collagen will help your skin glow and encourage fast healing.

Boosts Your Energy

Minerals and vitamins are good sources of energy for the body. Plants are not only rich in them, but also contain phytonutrients, antioxidants, proteins, and healthy fats. All of these are essential nutrients for your brain. In addition, they are easy to digest, which makes it easy for the body to obtain energy from them.

Lowers Blood Sugar Levels

The plant-based diet has little or no sugars at all. Most non-plant diets are known to contain high levels of sugars. This, in turn, causes diabetes. A plant-based diet lowers the level of blood sugar thereby making it healthy for your body.

Enhances Your Digestion

Good digestion calls for plenty of fiber. The good news is that plants offer sufficient fiber to facilitate good digestion. It is vital to understand that you cannot just start eating tons of vegetables and fruits without a plan. If you are starting this diet, you should start slow. Your body needs ample time to adjust. Therefore, you should introduce your new diet slowly to prevent constipation, since most of it is composed of fiber.

Prevents Chronic Diseases

Besides aiding in weight loss, a whole-food plant-based diet has also been proven to help lower the risks of various chronic health conditions.

Cardiac Conditions

This is the most widely-known benefit of whole-food plant-based diets as they have higher probabilities of keeping your cardiac health sound. But, the strength of this benefit is dependent on the types and quality of the food in your diet plan. Major research done on over 200,000 people concluded that the risk of having heart disease was lower in those people whose diet plan was plant-based and was rich in whole grains, veggies, nuts, legumes, and fruits than those who were following non-plant-based diets.

But, plant-based diet plans that are unhealthy because of the inclusion of fruit juices, refined grains, and sugary drinks showed an increased risk of cardiac complications. This is why it is very important to stick to the right foods and follow a healthy plant-based diet plan.

Cancer

According to various research studies, a plant-based diet plan can lower the risks of various forms of cancer. A study of over 69,000 people found that the risk of gastrointestinal cancer was very low for vegetarian diet followers, especially for Lacto-ovo vegetarian diet followers (the ones who consume both dairy and eggs).

In another study of over 77,000 people, it was proven that there was a 22 percent reduced risk of having colorectal cancer in those who followed a vegetarian diet plan than those who didn't. The safest was pescatarians (those vegetarians who consume fish) as they had a significant 43 percent lower risk of colorectal cancer than non-vegetarian diet plan followers.

Cognitive Decline

Various studies found that diet plans high in fruit and veggie content can prevent or slow Alzheimer's disease and cognitive decline in adults. The reason is that many foods in plant-based diet plans are high in antioxidants and plant compounds that act as protective agents against the development of Alzheimer's disease and reversing cognitive damage.

A review of nine research studies of around 31,000 people found that those who consumed more veggies and fruits had a significant 20 percent lower risk of having dementia or cognitive impairment.

Diabetes

A whole-food plant-based diet plan can play a significant role in lowering the risk of contracting diabetes or managing the illness. In a study involving over 200,000 people, it was proven that there was a 34 percent reduced risk of having diabetes if you followed a healthy, plant-based diet in comparison to an unhealthy, non-plant-based plan.

In another research study, it was proven that both Lacto-ovo vegetarian and vegan diet plans could lower the risk of type 2 diabetes by a whopping 50 percent in comparison to non-plant-based diet plans. Plant-based diet plans are also known to cause improvements in blood sugar level control in people with diabetes as compared to non-plant-based diets.

Saves Time and Money

A plant-based diet is generally known to be cheaper compared to a non-plant diet such as meat. When it also comes to cooking, a plant-based diet takes less time to be ready thereby saving you some valuable time which you can use to do other things.

Soothed Stomach

Eating too much meat, dairy, processed foods, and fatty foods, not chewing enough, and being under stress can all cause your stomach to act up and could be the culprit in heartburn and indigestion.

Faster Recovery After Workouts

Athletes, runners, and bodybuilders on plant-based diets report that they recover faster after workouts, meaning they can fit in more training than their omnivorous counterparts. This may be due to increased antioxidants, vitamins, potassium, or a decrease in the inflammatory compounds found in meat and dairy.

More Eco-Friendly Diet

The whole-food plant-based diet plan is not only beneficial in terms of health but also proven to be better for the ecosystem. Plant-based diet plan followers tend to have a smaller effect on the environment in comparison to other diet plan followers.

Sustainable eating approaches can help lower greenhouse gas effects as well as land and water consumption required for factory farming. These factors are known to be the major cause of harm to the ecosystem and global warming.

Around 64 different research studies found that diets with a minimal amount of animal-based foods like pescatarian, vegetarian, and vegan diet plans are known to be the most beneficial in terms of the environment. These studies also found that the transition of Western diet plans to a healthy, plant-based diet plan can result in 50 percent lower water usage and a significant 70 percent reduction in land usage and greenhouse gas emissions.

In addition to this, lowering animal-based food and choosing sustainable and locally-grown products can boost the economy and lower dependency on unsustainable practices like factory farming.

Chapter 3: The Plant-Based Diet

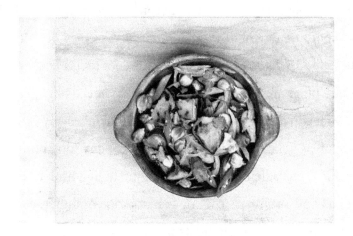

Differences with Other Diets

Vegetarian

A plant-based diet is totally different from a vegetarian diet. The main difference is that vegetarians eat some animal products such as honey and milk while a plant-based diet is exclusively made of plant products only.

Vegan

There has often been some confusion as to whether the plant-based diet is just another word for veganism, or if they are a completely different concept with different rules, so let's go into that. There are many similarities between the two, but also some distinct differences. Are veganism and a plant-based diet the same thing? The short answer is no. The particular diet that is chosen and the label it is given depends on the individual, and the reason they have chosen to live this lifestyle. Many vegans choose to be so because they disagree with the slaughter and poor treatment of farm animals, and so they do not consume these foods. They also usually choose not to use leather or wear fur or any other animal products. Vegans do not eat any sort of meat, or product containing traces of meat. This includes any broths or ingredients such as gelatin. Vegans also do not eat any food products that contain ANY ingredient from an animal, including milk or honey. They do not eat any cheese, or yogurt, or margarine or butter, etc. Some slightly more hidden ingredients that contain animal products are whey and casein. These are all avoided. Vegans get most of their food from plant sources, but they are not strictly whole food plant based. They may not be as health conscious, and so many may choose to eat packaged and processed foods, yet stay away from those made of animals. This technically still falls within the parameter of their diet.

Plant based folks eat a primarily plant derived diet- as close to nature as possible. But this does not mean that they are vegan, or even vegetarian. They may simply choose to eat mostly fruits, vegetables, nuts and legumes, etc. However, they may still choose to eat meat, and carefully choose meats that are antibiotics free, grass fed, and lived a free-range life. Many plant-based dieters believe that meat is still an integral part of a healthy diet, and so they just choose the best quality possible.

Whole food, plant-based diets usually take the qualities of both diets and even go a step further. Keeping foods whole refers to leaving them in their most natural state. So, vegetables and fruit are eaten as they are fresh, frozen or dried without preservatives or added flavor. Nuts are natural, without salt or sugar; grains are not refined or enriched or bleached. Most foods are prepared at home, or in a restaurant where the chefs share the same standards, as to not degrade any of the ingredients or take away any of their nutritional value. Many processed foods use what is known as plant fragments, rather than whole plants. They are reduced, or extracted or otherwise processed in some way.

Whatever the specifics of the diet someone chooses, if they tell you that they are vegan or plant based, you should assume that they do not consume any animal products at all, unless they mention it otherwise. This can help you to avoid accidentally serving them something that they will not be willing or able to eat. And feel free to ask someone about their diet, if you are curious. But make sure that they are willing to talk about it, and also that you listen with an open mind-not looking to judge or challenge their decision to adopt that particular diet.

Pescatarian

The pescatarians adhere to a diet with seafood as the sole meat source. It is clearly different from a plant-based diet because it incorporates seafood and eggs dairy products, which are not part of the plant-based diet. Pescatarians cannot eat other meat apart from seafood.

Flexitarian

A flexitarian usually eats a plant-based diet but occasionally adds meats to the diet. They are also known as semi-vegetarians.

Fruitarian

This is a veganism subset and it mainly or fully consists of fruits, seeds and nuts. It does not include animal products. The difference with the plant-based diet is that fruitarianism only considers fruits and seeds while a plant-based diet considers other plants as food.

Macrobiotic diet

This diet combines the concepts of principles of certain diets and spirituality of Buddhism to balance physical and spiritual wellness

The Plant-Based Food Group

Leaves

Leaf vegetables, or greens, are one of the most nutrient-dense foods you can eat. They contain plenty of vitamins (especially K, A, C, and folate) and minerals (like iron, magnesium, and potassium), as well as lots of chlorophyll, which is cleansing to the human system, particularly the liver. If you feel maxed out on salads, try adding some greens to a fruit smoothie or a soup. Puréed greens shrink quite a bit. The wide variety of leaves includes lettuce, kale, spinach, cabbage, Swiss chard, mizuna, arugula, bok choy, collard greens, mustard greens, dandelion greens, endive, escarole, watercress, sorrel, and tatsoi.

Roots

Root vegetables are generally made up of complex carbohydrates and starches. This is why they are usually cooked before being eaten, since cooking breaks down the starch molecules into easier-to-digest forms. However, carrots and radishes are commonly eaten raw in North America. The many root vegetables include carrot, beet, parsnip, rutabaga, turnip, sweet potato, potato, celeriac, and radish. Many root vegetables, such as beets, radishes, and turnips, also have very tasty leaves.

Bulbs

This group includes onions, leeks, and garlic. Garlic's claim to fame is boosting cardiovascular health; it's been shown in many studies to reduce cholesterol, inhibit platelet aggregation (when platelets in the blood stick together, which is how clots form), and reduce blood pressure. Onions are also recommended for cardiovascular health, since they have sulfur compounds similar to the ones that make garlic so powerful.

Stems

Stem vegetables include asparagus, celery, and kohlrabi. They are all very nutritious green vegetables with very few calories. Kohlrabi is a relative of cabbage and broccoli, so it contains the powerful cancer-fighting and anti-inflammatory compounds of this family of vegetables.

Vines

Although some of these vegetables are botanically considered fruit, when it comes to nutrition and cooking, they are in the vegetable category. These vegetables have high water content and will shrink considerably when cooked. Because this category includes a variety of vegetables, they have very different nutritional profiles, but vine veggies are generally rich in carotenoids and vitamin C. Vine vegetables include zucchini, squash, eggplant, cucumber, peas, okra, tomato, and bell and hot peppers.

Flowers

Yes, flowers can also be vegetables! This group includes broccoli, cauliflower, and artichoke. Broccoli, as a dark green vegetable, is packed with nutrients and antioxidants. Although cauliflower has no color, it has similar nutrients and is just as good for you like broccoli.

Mushrooms

Mushrooms are not plants (they are fungi), but nutritionally they get lumped in with vegetables. The difference with mushrooms is that they eat organic matter and do not use photosynthesis like plants. Since they are a totally different organism than other vegetables, they have value in our diet by bringing in different nutrients, such as selenium and copper, as well as a powerful anti-inflammatory, cardioprotective, cancer-protective, and immune-supportive compounds. Mushrooms are high in minerals and protein per calorie and are also a good source of B vitamins.

Some of the mushrooms you might find in your local markets include chanterelle, shiitake, oyster, cremini, button, morel, and puffball. There are also many other types of edible mushrooms, including mushrooms used for their healing powers in Chinese medicine—some powerful enough to combat cancer.

Nuts and seeds

1.   Chia Seeds

Chia seeds are amazing sources of vitamin C, protein, fiber, and calcium. They have to be soaked in liquid and allowed to expand.

Once properly prepared, you can sprinkle them on top of almost anything!

2.   Pumpkin Seeds

Pumpkin seeds work great for a tasty and easy snack and can also be added to salads, yogurt, and soups. They pack a lot of great nutrients like Vitamins C, E, and K, omega-3 fatty acids, and iron in a small package.

3.   Almonds

Commonly considered nuts, almonds are more accurately categorized as a fruit of the almond tree. They are wonderful sources of fiber, protein, magnesium, phosphorus, calcium, potassium, iron, and B vitamins. Like soybeans, they are often used in dairy substitutes and they have been shown to lower cholesterol, strengthen bones, and promote a healthy cardiovascular system. Plus, they are great for your skin and hair!

4.   Flaxseeds

Flaxseeds are great additives to plant-based meals. They can be ground up and added to smoothies, oatmeal, cereal, or baked into muffins, bread, and cookies. They are high in protein, magnesium, zinc, and B vitamins. They also aid in digestion and help with weight loss by suppressing appetite.

5.   Walnuts

These nuts are some of the best natural sources of omega-3 fatty acids.
They also contain plenty of vitamin E, protein, calcium, zinc, and
potassium. These, like many of the other nuts and seeds on this list,
can be enjoyed alone as a snack or added to other dishes.

6.   Sesame Seeds

Sesame seeds are a great natural way to lower cholesterol and high
blood pressure and can also help with afflictions like migraines,
arthritis, and asthma. They are great in bread and crackers and can be
used in stir-fry meals and salads.

7.   Sunflower Seeds

These seeds are great for vitamin E and contain healthy fats, B
vitamins, and iron. They can be eaten dry and are also used to make
butter, a great alternative to dairy.

8.   Cashews

Though cashews, like almonds, are not technically nuts and are rather
the fruit of the cashew tree, they are most commonly treated as nuts.
With their low sodium content and great flavor, they are a popular
source of protein and vitamins.

9.   Brazil Nuts

These delicious nuts from the Bertholletia excelsa tree mature inside a large coconut-like shell. They are wonderful for protein, fiber, iron, and many B-complex vitamins.

10.   Pine Nuts

Pine nuts contain great antioxidants as well as lots of iron, magnesium, and potassium. They are low in calories and go wonderfully with many dishes. You can use them in baked foods or add them in sauces like an Italian pesto.

Legumes

1.   Edamame

These cooked soybeans are not only delicious, but they also have an incredible amount of protein. In just one cup, a serving of edamame will give you 18 grams of protein. Look for the certified organic seal, though, because many soybeans in the United States are treated with pesticides or genetically modified. Edamame works great as a stand-alone snack or appetizer and can also be added into meals as a side or in a stir-fry.

2.   Lentils

Easy to incorporate into almost any meal in a variety of forms, lentils provide an excellent source of low-calorie and high-fiber protein. They contain 9 grams of protein per half cup serving. They are also incredibly helpful in lowering cholesterol and promoting heart health. You can prepare them as a side dish, use them to make veggie burgers, substitute them for meat and make a delicious taco filling in a slow cooker or make a yummy dip with them.

3.   Black Beans

Black beans are another vegetable like lentils that are wonderfully multi-use. They have great fiber, folate, potassium, and vitamin B6. They contain 7.6 grams of protein in every serving and can be used to make anything from veggie burgers to vegan brownies. Imagine that!

4.   Potatoes

Potatoes are a great, low-cost source of protein (4 grams per medium potato) and potassium. They're tasty and heart-healthy!

5.   Spinach

One of the best green vegetables for protein (3 grams per serving), cooked spinach is an excellent addition to your plant-based diet.

6.   Broccoli

When cooked, you get 2 grams per serving of this vegetable and also an excellent dose of fiber.

7.   Brussels Sprouts

Another great green vegetable for protein, Brussels sprouts gives you 2 grams of protein per serving alongside a great deal of potassium and vitamin K. Be sure to get the fresh version, though, as they taste a whole lot better than the frozen kind!

8.   Lima Beans

Containing 7.3 grams of protein per serving when cooked, lima beans make an amazing side dish or addition to a healthy salad. They also contain leucine, an amino acid that aids in muscle synthesis!

9.   Peanuts and Peanut Butter

Widely recognized as a super food by meat-eaters and plant-based eaters alike, peanuts and peanut butter contain 7 grams of protein per serving and can be used in so many different ways. And who doesn't love a good childhood staple PB&J sandwich? Nearly all kinds of peanut butter are vegan, but keep a lookout for any that might contain honey if you are keeping strictly vegan and cutting out all animal products.

10.   Chickpeas

Chickpeas are another versatile legume that can be prepared in a multitude of ways. Perhaps the most popular preparation is in the form of delicious hummus. With 6 grams of protein per serving, it'll be hard not to spread it on everything you eat!

Whole Grains

1.   Quinoa

Quinoa certainly has made a splash onto the health food scene with countless people boasting about its beneficial qualities. Although it is actually a seed, we treat it mainly as a grain in the way in which it is prepared. This South American gem has an incredible amount of protein and omega-3 fatty acids and is an important staple of anyone looking to get more of these nutrients within a plant-based diet. It can be used in a multitude of dishes and is as versatile as it is healthy!

2.   Wheat

A classic staple, whole wheat is incredibly beneficial to your health. Each serving of whole grain has about 2 to 3 grams of fiber, which is a great way to make sure your body is functioning healthily and properly. Be sure to steer clear of multi-grain, however, and go for the stuff marked 100% whole grain to make sure you are getting exactly what you need!

3.   Oats

These whole grains are packed full of heart-healthy antioxidants. Oats are great and can be enjoyed as a fulfilling breakfast in the form of oatmeal and they can also be ground up and used as a healthier flour substitute when baking. Unsweetened oats are the best to buy and if you are craving a little something sugary, throw in a few berries or a dollop of honey if you wish.

4.   Brown Rice

Brown rice is incredibly high in antioxidants and good vitamins. It is relative, white rice is far less beneficial as much of these healthy nutrients get destroyed during the process of milling. You can also opt for red and black rice or wild rice. The meal options for this healthy grain are limitless!

5.   Rye

Rye is an amazing whole grain that contains four times the fiber of regular whole wheat and gives you almost 50% of day-to-day recommended iron intake. When shopping for rye, however, be sure to look for the whole rye marking as a lot of what is on the market is made with refined flour, thus cutting the benefits in half.

6.   Barley

This whole grain is a miracle food for lowering high cholesterol. It can be quick-cooked like oats and serves as a delicious side dish. You can add whatever kind of toppings you desire to give it your own personal flair! Be sure again to seek out the whole-grain barley as other types may have the bran or germ removed.

7.   Buckwheat

Buckwheat is a great gluten-free grain option for those with celiac disease or gluten intolerance. It's a great source of magnesium and manganese. Buckwheat is used to make delicious gluten free pancakes and easily becomes a morning staple!

8.   Bulgur

This grain is a truly excellent source of iron and magnesium. It also contains a wonderful amount of protein and fiber with one cup containing about 75% of daily recommended fiber and 25% or daily recommended protein. It goes great in salads and soups and is easy to cook. Talk about amazing!

9.   Couscous

This grain is another great source of fiber. A lot of the couscous you see in the store will be made from refined flour, though, so you must seek out the whole wheat kind so that you can get all the healthy, yummy benefits.

10.   Corn

Whole corn is a fantastic source of phosphorus, magnesium, and B vitamins. It also promotes healthy digestion and contains heart-healthy antioxidants. It is important to seek out organic corn in order to bypass all of the genetically modified product that is out on the market.

Fruits

1.   Avocado

Widely acknowledged as an incredibly beneficial and healthy super-fruit, avocados truly are miracle fruits. They are the best way possible to get the kind of substantial serving of healthy monounsaturated fatty acids that many people subscribing to a plant-based diet seek to supplement. They also contain about 20 different vitamins and minerals and are packed with important nutrients. On top of that, they taste amazing and go well with almost any dish, breakfast, lunch, or dinner!

2.   Grapefruit

Grapefruits are packed full of Vitamin C, containing much more than oranges. Half a grapefruit provides you with almost 50% of your recommended daily vitamin C. It also gives you incredible levels of Vitamin A, fiber, and potassium. It can help with afflictions like arthritis and is a great remedy for oily skin.

3.   Pineapple

This fruit can be prepared and enjoyed in a variety of ways making it not only a tasty and fun treat but also a great healthy choice! It is full of anti-inflammatory nutrients that can help reduce the risk of stroke or heart attack. Some studies show that it also increases fertility.

4.   Blueberries

These little berries not only taste delicious and go with so many different dishes, but they are also full of vitamin C and healthful antioxidants. Studies also show that it promotes eye health and can slow macular degeneration, which causes older adults to go blind.

5.   Pomegranate

Whether in juice form or seed, consuming pomegranate is a great way to get potassium. It has fantastic antioxidants (three times more than green tea or red wine) that work to promote cardiovascular and heart health as well as lower cholesterol levels

6.   Apple

The old saying "an apple a day keeps the doctor away" is not just an old wife' tale! It is low-calorie and incredibly healthy. Apples contain antioxidants that protect brain cell health and are heart-healthy. They can also lower high cholesterol and aid in weight loss and healthy teeth.

7.   Kiwi

This tart, delicious fruit is not only unique but also full of great vitamins like C and E. These are powerful antioxidants that some studies show help with eye health and can even lower the chances of cancer. They are low-calorie and very high in fiber. This makes them great for aiding in weight loss and they make a wonderful, quick, easy, and guilt-free snack.

8.   Mango

Mangoes have excellent levels of the nutrient beta-carotene. The body converts this into Vitamin A, which in turn strengthens bone health and the immune system. They also have a huge amount of Vitamin C- 50% of the daily recommended value to be exact.

9.   Lemons

Everyone knows that lemons and other citrus fruit are high in Vitamin C, however, they are also an excellent source of antioxidants, fiber, and folate. Lemons can help lower cholesterol, the risk of some kinds of cancer, and blood pressure. All at just 17 calories a serving!

10.   Cranberries

Cranberries are another fruit that has more than one health benefit. They have great vitamin C and fiber levels and have more antioxidants than many other fruits and vegetables. At only 45 calories a serving, it is a great way to boost your immune system, keep your urinary tract healthy, and absorb other important nutrients like Vitamins E, K, and manganese.

Spices and Herbs

Spices and herbs are not only a way to add rich flavor to your dishes but they also have small amounts of important nutrients. A study of vegetarian males eating an Indian diet showed that they got between 3.9 and 7.9 percent of their essential amino acid requirements, along with about 6 percent of calcium and 4 percent of iron, just from the seasonings in their food.

Many spices have protein, and although it doesn't amount to much in terms of grams, it provides a source of some of the amino acids that may be low in plant foods. Popular spices that will add a world of flavor to your food include cumin, coriander, cinnamon, paprika, and nutmeg.

Herbs like parsley, cilantro, mint, ginger, and basil pack loads of nutrients, and are most beneficial and flavorful when you eat them fresh. Parsley gives women 22 percent of their daily vitamin C recommendation, and men 27 percent, in just 4 tablespoons. All fresh herbs, like leafy greens, have a high antioxidant and chlorophyll content, providing energy and helping your body neutralize free radicals.

Nutrients in Plant-Based Diet

Carbohydrates

Some people worry about consuming too many carbohydrates by eating plant foods. Carbohydrates are your body's main source of energy and are completely healthy if you eat them in the form of whole foods (such as whole grains, vegetables, and fruit), since they contain lots of vitamins, minerals, antioxidants, water, and fiber. Fiber is also a carbohydrate, but its role is to facilitate digestion rather than give energy.

Whole grains and fruit have the highest levels of carbohydrates, with about 70 to 90 percent carbohydrate content. Eating a banana is an instant energy boost. The best food sources of fiber are psyllium or flaxseed and leafy green vegetables.

Protein

Protein can be found in all cells of the body. It helps to repair and build muscles, skin, bones, and the immune system. Protein is also needed to create hormones and enzymes, which are made up of amino acids. The body can make some of the amino acids but definitely not all of them. The ones the body can't make are called essential amino acids and must come from the foods you eat. Eating mostly plant-based foods can meet your body's daily protein needs.

Protein is an essential nutrient in the body. It not only helps in building and repairing muscles, but it also aids in maintaining our skin and bone health. The immune system also requires protein to function optimally in warding off diseases. So, if you are new to a vegan diet, you may have questions concerning your protein sources. Of course, this is attributed to the myth that plant-based diets don't provide the body with sufficient nutrients.

However, several plant foods will provide you with the protein you need in your diet. Some of these foods include beans, soy products, seeds, nuts, peas, vegetables, and whole grains. When looking for proteins in vegetables, your shopping cart should be filled with veggies like broccoli, yellow sweet corn, potatoes, lentils, green peas, Brussels sprouts, broccoli rabe, avocado, and cauliflower.

Evidently, you can see that you have plenty of options to choose from when in search of protein in your diet. Now, let's do some math to determine the amount of protein you might need in your diet. According to the Dietary Reference Intakes, the amount of protein you should consume daily is equivalent to 0.8 grams per kilogram of your body weight, or 0.36 grams per pound. Say you weigh 80 kilograms. You should multiply this by 0.8 grams to determine the protein quantity you require daily. In this case, the quantity of protein will be 64 grams.

The various foods mentioned above offer varying amounts of protein. This implies that combining several veggies together will provide you with what you need. A one cup serving of lentils, for instance, will provide you with 18 grams of protein. A cup of green peas, on the other hand, will only provide you with 8.5 grams of protein. Judging from the numbers, all you need is a mix of different plant foods to meet your daily protein intake.

Fats

Your body needs enough dietary fat to function, maintain metabolism, and absorb and utilize minerals and certain vitamins. People with cold hands and feet, amenorrhea (missed menstrual periods), or dry skin, hair, or throat may need more fats in their diet, and particularly saturated fats like coconut oil. To be clear, eating healthy fat in reasonable amounts doesn't make you fat.

The best source of healthy fat is whole plant foods—avocados, nuts, and seeds (including nut and seed butter). These average about 80 percent fat. Whole grains and beans also have some healthy fat, and there are even small amounts in fruits, vegetables, spices, and pretty much every food. Oats, for example, are about 15 percent fat.

Oils are 100 percent fat and aren't something you necessarily need to eat, but they are great for carrying rich flavor and mouthfeel in a dish, particularly when you're transitioning to a healthier diet. If you use oils, it's best to keep them minimal and use unrefined oils like olive, coconut, sesame, and avocado. (Refined oils include canola, soy, sunflower, and corn oil.) You can easily sauté vegetables for two people with just a teaspoon of oil.

That doesn't mean you should never eat oils, though, and some people can actually benefit from concentrated fats. For example, flax oil or concentrated DHA might be necessary for someone with issues digesting and utilizing omega-3 fatty acids.

Omega-3 fatty acids are also essential nutrients, meaning that the body cannot produce them. There are three forms of omega-3 fatty acids:

- Docosahexaenoic acid (DHA)

- Alpha-linolenic acid (ALA)

- Eicosapentaenoic acid (EPA)

Individuals who eat fish usually obtain DHA and EPA. ALA, on the other hand, is obtained from plant foods. The good news is that the body can convert ALA obtained from plants into DHA and EPA. However, the process is not as efficient. Consequently, you could supplement your diet with hemp seed oil, flaxseed oil, or chia seeds to aid in optimizing the conversion process.

Other recommended foods to ingest include algal oil, walnuts, perilla oil, and Brussels sprouts.

The information detailed in this section should help you realize that important nutrients that are often assumed to be present only in animal products can also be obtained from plant foods. Therefore, knowing and understanding the nutrients you are getting from your plant foods is important; it confirms that you are getting all the vital nutrients your body requires for optimal functioning.

Vitamins

Vitamin C

Vitamin C will be an easier nutrient to obtain since most fruits and vegetables can provide the body with this vital nutrient. This vitamin helps in strengthening the body's immune system. As a result, vitamin C is often perceived as a remedy for the common cold. Recommended vegan foods to add to your diet here include broccoli, pineapple, Brussels sprouts, kiwi, bell peppers, oranges, and spinach. All of these foods provide you with varying quantities of vitamin C. For instance, a one cup serving of broccoli will provide you with about 81 mg of vitamin C. A higher quantity can be gained from a cup of kiwi since it provides you with nearly 167 mg of the nutrient (Von Alt, 2017).

Vitamin B12

Like iron, vitamin B12 is an essential nutrient required for the optimal functioning of the brain. Additionally, it helps in the production of red blood cells. The vitamin can be found in fortified foods including cereals, nutritional yeast, hemp milk, and meat substitutes. Before purchasing these products from the stores, you must read the nutrition labels. This way, you avoid taking home foods high in sugar and other unhealthy oils.

Mineral salts

Iron

There are various functions of iron in our bodies. This makes this nutrient very important. The nutrient is required for blood production. It also aids in the transportation of oxygen in the blood through the production of hemoglobin. Lack of iron in the blood will result in the body not obtaining sufficient oxygen. The presence of iron in the body also guarantees that the food we eat is easily converted into energy (Spatone, "What Does Iron Do for the Body? The Role of Iron: Spatone"). It is also worth mentioning that the body requires iron for optimal cognitive function. Brain functions that depend on iron include alertness, attention, memory, intelligence, problem-solving, and learning. Therefore, a balanced intake of iron ensures that our brains function well.

The above-mentioned benefits of iron prove that iron is indeed an important nutrient that the body requires. Unfortunately, the body doesn't naturally produce iron. Consequently, it is up to us to supplement it through good food choices. Plant foods that provide us with iron include legumes, nuts and seeds, grains, and vegetables.

Ideal legumes to shop for are lentils, tofu, lima beans, chickpeas, black beans, and soybeans. The best grains to shop for here include fortified cereals, oatmeal, brown rice, and quinoa. In terms of nuts and seeds, you should go for pine, squash, pumpkin, sunflower, cashews, and pistachios. Collard greens, Swiss chard, and tomato sauce are also excellent sources of iron in the vegetable category.

Calcium

When you think of calcium, the first thing that comes to mind is milk, right? Well, over the years, we have been made to understand that dairy foods are the best sources of calcium. While this is true, you should also realize that the nutrient can be obtained from plant foods. To avoid the negative health effects associated with dairy and other animal products, it is best to choose certain plant foods.

Calcium is of great importance to our bone health and teeth development. It also has a role to play in nerve signaling, muscle function, and heart health. Adults should ingest 1,000 mg of calcium daily. Children should have an even higher intake of 1,300 mg daily (Jennings, 2018).

Ideal plant-based sources of calcium include bok choy, Chinese cabbage, broccoli, calcium-set tofu, beans, lentils, and fruits. The best fruits here include blackberries, blackcurrants, and raspberries.

Zinc

Zinc has several important functions in the body. It is ranked as an essential nutrient because the body cannot naturally produce it. Hence, it is worth knowing how you can supplement your diet to ensure that you provide your body with this nutrient. Zinc comes second as the most abundant mineral in the body after iron. The mineral helps with metabolism, nerve function, digestion, and immune functions.

So, which foods should you eat to get zinc? Ideal sources include tempeh, whole grains, tofu, lentils, seeds, nuts, peas, beans, and several fortified kinds of cereals. In some cases, the body due to phytates compounds might not easily absorb zinc. Therefore, it is highly recommended that you soak some of these foods before cooking. Grains, seeds, and beans fall into this category.

Chloride

This mineral plays a part in body fluid balance including digestive juices. It is found in sea salt, tomatoes, lettuce, celery, and rye bread.

Magnesium

This mineral regulates blood sugar and assists in energy production. It also helps your muscles, kidneys, bones and heart function effectively. It is found in spinach, quinoa, dark chocolate, almonds, avocado, and black beans.

Phosphorous

This mineral is found in bones and works with calcium in maintaining healthy mineral balance within the body. It is found in pumpkin, sunflower seeds, lentils, chickpeas, oatmeal, and quinoa.

Sodium

The current population gets excess sodium from all pre-packaged foods and restaurant meals, so there is no need to go looking for extra sodium in the diet.

Potassium

This mineral is essential in blood pressure balance, muscle health, and nerve function. It is found in avocado, bananas, apricots, grapefruit, potatoes, mushrooms, cucumbers and zucchini.

Plant-Based Diet: Common Myths

The first thing that might come to your mind when you think of a plant-based diet is that it is quite limited and unhealthy. This is what many people tend to think because of their lack of information. They are not fully aware of the fact that a plant-based diet is not nutrient-deficient as they may think. About this, there are several myths in regards to this diet that you may come across.

Diet Lacks Enough Calcium

Calcium is certainly beneficial to our bodies. It not only aids in strengthening our bones, but it also guarantees optimal muscle and nerve function. Besides this, it also helps in blood clotting. Keeping this in mind, it is crucial to make sure that you aren't lacking this nutrient in your diet. Unfortunately, most people have the assumption that plant-based foods lack calcium because there is an absence of milk. What they fail to understand is that milk isn't the only reliable source of calcium.

When sticking to a plant-based diet, non-dairy foods that will provide plenty of calcium include oranges, fortified nut milk, tofu, and dark green vegetables. The list doesn't end here; other alternatives to include in your diet are soybeans, Chinese cabbage, collards, mustard greens, bok choy, and broccoli (Hansard, 2017).

When shopping for your veggies, check the product labels to determine the amount of calcium you will be getting from your food. With time, you will realize that it is quite easy to obtain calcium from vegetables, contrary to what most people believe.

Meat Is the Main Source of Protein

You will also come across stories from many people claiming that meat is the main source of protein. Sure, meat provides us with proteins, but there are plenty of other protein sources out there. In fact, only fats and fruits lack proteins. The rest of the foods that we eat provide us with protein nutrients. This means that, if you are eating a diverse range of foods, then you can be sure that you are not missing protein nutrients.

Some veggies that are rich in protein include kale, collards, and spinach. Later on, you will notice that these foods are included in most of the recipes we provide in the book. An important note to bear in mind when consuming vegetables is what is termed as alkaloid buildup. These are toxins present in all leafy greens. You should always rotate the consumption of your greens to make sure that these toxins don't build up.

Protein source alternatives include soy products, nuts, whole grains, legumes, and seeds. The best thing about these plant-based foods is that they not only provide you with proteins, but they ensure you consume fewer saturated fats and plenty of fiber. Therefore, your overall good health is maintained.

Plant-Based Diets Are Costly

With the wide range of plants that you have to choose from, you might end up believing that a plant-based diet is expensive to maintain. Most people believe this is true. However, this is not the case. Just like any other diet, you need to plan for your meals. This necessitates you sticking to your budget and saving money while shopping.

When buying fruits and veggies, it is advisable to settle for ingredients that can be frozen. This prevents you from having to shop frequently. More importantly, if you live close to farming areas, you should take advantage of local farm products as they are affordable. Another crucial thing to remember is that some vegetables and fruits are high in pesticides. Stick to organic products to avoid these harmful chemicals. Foods that fall into this category include potatoes, lettuce, green beans, celery, apples, peaches, spinach, kale, and cucumbers.

Some foods that you don't have to go organic with include sweet corn, avocado, sweet potatoes, watermelon, sweet peas, pineapples, onions, mangoes, kiwi, and grapefruit.

Plant-Based Diets Are Not Ideal for Children, Athletes, or Pregnant Women

A huge misconception about plant-based diets is that they lack sufficient nutrients to help children grow or to aid pregnant women in supporting their unborn child while still supporting themselves. Also, some athletes might develop a similar misunderstanding. This, however, is not true as the diet can provide all the nutrients required to live a healthy life. The best part is that the diet eliminates all kinds of unhealthy meats that may have negative effects.

Products Labeled "Vegetarian" Are Healthy

Now that you want to try the plant-based diet, you should be careful with what you choose to buy. There are products which will be labeled "vegetarian," but are not as healthy as you think. From the previous definition of a plant-based diet, you should understand that most of your foods should be whole foods that are minimally processed. The issue with processed products is that some have high oil and sugar content. So, when you find a vegetarian product while shopping, check the label carefully to make sure that you are taking home a low-sugar, low-fat, low-sodium product.

Tips for Eating Plant-Based Out

One of the main reasons why new plant-based eaters end up quitting their diet program is because of the notion that they stand out from other people. You cannot avoid the fact that you will be eating out from time to time. Nonetheless, this might be a huge challenge for you if you are brand new to your plant-based diet. So, what should you do when you are dining out? Should you just eat because most of your friends are forcing you to do so? Or should you eat animal products because the restaurant lacks plant-based options?

Truly, it can be challenging to eat out if you are trying out a new diet. It might affect the goals that you initially had. The worst case is that it might even end up affecting your overall outlook towards going plant-based diet. The good news is that there are numerous restaurants today which offer plant-based dishes. However, this will not prevent you from being inquisitive about the way in which the meals were prepared. If you are strict on being plant-based, you will want to know whether the right types of oils were used in preparing the meals. In fact, you might even muster the courage to ask the chefs if it is possible to modify the food a little bit.

The challenging experience of dining in restaurants can, at times, make you feel as though you are too demanding. Your social circle might also think the same of you. What they don't understand is that you are trying to develop a habit, and it takes time to create a routine that you can easily stick to. The following sections will outline ideal tips that you should consider when eating plant foods at restaurants.

Plan Ahead

You can't always be sure that you will be dining at restaurants that offer a good plant-based diet. Therefore, you need to plan ahead for this trip. Before going out to a particular restaurant, start by checking their menu online. This gives you early information about whether the restaurant offers options that you are looking for. There are instances when these dishes will not be present. However, if you look closely, some foods can be made plant-based. For instance, removing chicken from well-cooked veggies might make a huge difference.

Call Ahead

If there is nothing plant-based you found in a restaurant menu, this doesn't mean that you should settle for anything. Frankly, you will be nervous to eat anything since you are cautious about your diet. So, you need to call the restaurant ahead of time and ask them. If they don't have what you are looking for, you can easily make changes early enough without inconveniencing anyone.

The idea of calling ahead is indeed helpful, more so when you are eating out with friends, family, or colleagues. Since restaurants will want to create a lasting impression, some of them may offer to prepare a small vegetarian meal for you. Therefore, you can relax knowing that you don't have to pick apart their menu when you arrive.

Ask for Modifications

It is also not a bad idea to ask whether some modifications can be made to your meal. There are some vegetarian diets that can easily be changed into plant-based by replacing one or two things. For instance, using oil instead of butter and getting rid of cheese can make a huge difference to the meal.

If you are going to make special requests, it is crucial that you ask politely. This is the best and most considerate way in which you will get the chefs to listen to you. You need to realize that they are busy serving many people. If you talk rudely or come across as entitled or demanding, they might be less than eager to accommodate your request.

Eat Beforehand

If you do your research and realize that you have limited options, you could choose to eat before going out. This way, you won't have to eat anything at the restaurant. You can settle for drinks as you catch up with your close friends and relatives.

Use Mobile Apps

The advent of technology has really transformed the way we do things. You don't have to go from one restaurant to the other asking whether they have plant-based dishes. All you have to do is use mobile apps that can give you info on the best restaurants near you. You should also take advantage of these applications to locate ideal eateries with plant-based foods.

Don't Sweat It

If you know that the plant-based-friendly eateries around you are few and far between, then you shouldn't sweat it. Instead of focusing too much on what you are going to eat, center your attention on the experience you will be getting. This means believing that you will have a great time with friends and family. This is more fulfilling than stuffing yourself with the food you are not sure of.

Dining out when you are new to a plant-based diet can be challenging. Some people may view you differently. Some will not understand why you are choosing a meal that is, at least to them, less tasty. At some point, others might even ask you whether you are sick.

Weight Loss with Plant-Based Diet

If you have tried losing weight before, then you can attest to the fact that it is never an easy process. With the numerous weight loss diet plans out there, it is easy to get confused about what you should actually eat. This is where everything gets frustrating as you end up trying different forms of diets and nothing seems to work. Have you ever been there before? If so, this chapter strives to help you realize that a plant-based diet might be the best alternative for you. Besides, by losing weight naturally, there are tons of other health benefits you will gain.

Maybe you are already on a plant-based diet and you are concerned that you are not shedding any pounds. This is a common dilemma faced by many dieters. The following are some of the main reasons why you may be finding it difficult to lose weight while on a plant-based diet.

Eating Large Portions

Before pointing fingers at the diets that you are eating, you should consider whether you are eating the right portion sizes. The mere fact that you are eating plant foods only doesn't mean that your body will not respond to large portions. It is important to understand that, when eating veg-friendly diets, you will be supplying your body with all the essential nutrients that it requires. This means that providing more than enough is not advisable. Too many carbs, for example, will not help you lose weight in any way.

Therefore, you should reduce your portions to guarantee that you lose weight. Depending on your weight and height, there are specific foods that you will have to eat more compared to others. You cannot eat the exact same diet as your friend and expect the same results.

Eating Less Protein

Another possible reason why you are not losing weight on your plant-based diet is because your protein intake is inadequate. Try to rotate your meals by adding in some of the best plant foods that are rich sources of protein. They include quinoa, almonds, peanuts, chickpeas, lentils, and tofu, among others. Use the plate method to make sure that you are getting enough of these proteins. Alternatively, you can create a chart that defines the best protein sources for every meal you prepare. It might sound silly, but at the end of the day, you will be eating right and helping yourself to cut weight.

Poor Timing

Have you thought of your meal timing? If your meal timing is off, then you can be sure that you will gain weight instead of losing. For example, grabbing your largest meal at the end of the day is not advisable. In the evening, you should simply snack since you will be going to sleep. During this time, the body is least active and is in a resting state. Therefore, you don't have to eat to fill your belly in the evening.

Plant-Based Junk

You might not be losing weight because your plant-based foods consist of junk. Some folks assume that treating themselves to sweet potato chips or coconut milk ice cream will not harm. Unfortunately, these foods are still high in calories. Eating them once in a while is not bad, but snacking on them often will only result in you packing on the pounds. This will only frustrate you because you thought that you were eating healthily. Instead of consuming processed plant-based foods, ensure that you settle for whole foods that are fresh and nutrient-dense.

Drinking Your Calories

A huge problem with manufacturers today is that they care less about your health. As such, they will market anything which is profitable to them without putting any consideration on your health. There are some products that you might have fallen for, including coconut water, chia drinks, and green juices. If you check the labels closely, some of these drinks are high in calories. Hence, it will be difficult for you to lose weight if you drink them frequently. Sadly, some manufacturers are not honest with their packaging. You should try your best to blend juices from natural fruits. This way, you know what you are putting into your body.

Now, since you are aware of the main reasons why you might not be losing weight on a plant-based diet, let's get a deeper understanding of how you can lose weight effectively on a plant-based diet.

Transition Slowly

The first step that you take while adopting a new plant-based diet will make a huge difference in your weight loss goal. If you try to make quick changes, then there is a good chance that you will be back to your old habits in no time. Try to transition gradually. Start by ditching some of the animal products slowly before you replace them completely with plant alternatives. Give yourself time and set small goals each day. With time, your body will have fully adjusted and you will not crave animal-based foods anymore.

Don't Skip Meals

The idea of losing weight often pushes people to skip meals with the perception that they are helping their bodies slim down. However, since you are on a plant-only diet, you need to realize that you will require more food to meet the recommended daily calorie intake. Consequently, this means that you will have to eat breakfast, lunch, and dinner at the right times.

Instead of skipping meals, shuffle your meals to ensure that you eat foods that are rich in fiber. These dishes will keep you satiated and will prevent you from having to snack each time your cravings shoot up. Starving yourself is not part of a healthy, plant-based diet plan.

Meet Your Protein Intake

A key strategy for losing weight is to ensure that your metabolism is revved up. This is why it is beneficial that you meet your daily protein intake. Don't be fooled into thinking that plant-based foods will not meet your daily protein requirement. A lot has been discussed about this, so it should be easy for you to settle for the best plant foods that are considered ideal protein sources.

Start with a Salad

A clever tactic to lose weight while sticking to plant foods is to eat a salad before lunch and dinner. The main reason why this strategy works is because you provide your body with essential minerals and vitamins in your everyday meal. It also means that your stomach will be filled with fiber before grabbing your main meal course. Since you will feel satiated, there is a good chance that you will not overeat. In a way, you will naturally cut your portions. This sounds easy, right? With the simple tactic of adding a salad before eating your lunch or dinner, your overeating habit will be well-managed.

Spice Things up

It is highly recommended that you add spices and herbs to your cooking. You may have heard that chili peppers help with weight loss. Well, it is true. They contain capsaicin, a compound that helps in appetite suppression (Wong, 2018). The compound also aids in reducing fat tissue and, at the same time, speeding up your metabolism. Spicing things up will therefore help you meet your short- and long-term goals of slimming down.

Embrace Batch Cooking

Usually, we are forced to order food because we have tight schedules that we need to maintain. This stands as one of the main reasons why people find themselves eating junk food that ultimately contributes to

71

rapid weight gain. To save yourself from unhealthy eating habits, you must value the importance of batch cooking. This is the idea of cooking food in plenty and refrigerating or freezing it. The benefit here is that the leftover food will deter you from snacking. Eventually, you will maintain a healthy, balanced diet all throughout the week or month. You should expect positive waistline results if you maintain this habit for several months.

Stay Hydrated

Your body needs water to function optimally. Therefore, it should be obvious that you need to stay hydrated throughout the day. In addition to drinking plenty of water, you should eat a lot of fruit.

Be Consistent

The best way to lose weight over the long haul is to be consistent in eating right. The last thing that you should do is settle for a diet plan that you can only manage to stick to for a few weeks. It is important that you choose a plan that can last you months before thinking of anything else. This means that you should try to make your diet as interesting as possible.

Gaining momentum on your weight loss plan will depend on whether you are consistent with your eating habits or not. This calls for healthy diet choices every time. If you know that your workplace environment doesn't provide healthy dishes, prepare yourself a veg-friendly meal and carry it with you. Put in every effort towards losing weight by following your plan.

Keep It Simple

In conjunction with what has been said about consistency, you should keep your diet plan simple. Don't complicate things as this will only discourage you when you are not in the mood to cook or follow a particular diet. A great way of following your plan is by choosing the best plant dishes that you are interested in. In fact, this is crucial during your transition period since you are looking for an easier way to enjoy your meal while losing weight at the same time.

Plant-Based Diet Challenges

The commanding cultural norm for people living in the west is meat consumption. Most people in Western countries claim that they are trying to cut down on their meat consumption. However, according to statistics, this is not the case. According to the United States Department of Agriculture (USDA), there has been a rise in meat consumption over the past few years (Ritchie, 2019). Meat consumption is indeed beneficial. However, this only applies when eaten in moderate quantities. Unfortunately, most people over-consume meat far beyond what the body requires. This is what leads to health complications such as an increased risk for cancer and heart disease.

Information is spreading far and wide and people are beginning to realize that animal-based foods are only causing more harm than good to their lives. Other people are going the vegan way as they acknowledge that these animals should be protected. Whatever reasons you have for switching to plant foods, you should realize that you are outnumbered. As such, you should be ready to face the mental and physical challenges associated with plant-only diets. Some of these challenges and ideal solutions are succinctly discussed in this section.

Uninteresting Food

If you are switching to a new, plant-based diet, then you will face the challenge of perceiving your food as bland. You cannot blame yourself for feeling this way. It happens to most people since they are just transitioning from eating junk foods filled with sugar and other additives. So, expect your first dishes to seem boring. Considering the fact that there are many health benefits of plant-based dishes, you will want to find a way of bringing some excitement to your foods.

The good news is that there are plenty of ways to have fun while enjoying plant-based diets. For instance, you could mix things up with the many recipes that you can choose from. This guarantees that you never get tired of trying new things in the kitchen.

You Don't Long for Food

Another problem that you could face is that you might not have a strong desire for plant foods as compared to animal foods. The food cravings that you once had were simply because your body had been used to them. With the changes that you will be making to your diet, you shouldn't be surprised that you don't crave plant-based foods immediately. Avoid this by trying to understand that you are moving towards a healthier direction. It might not be easy, but eventually, it will pay off.

Social Settings Challenge

At times you will notice that it is difficult to feel comfortable in social settings where most people are not vegans or vegetarians. A rule of thumb you should always remember in such circumstances is that you should never lead by saying that you only eat a plant-based diet. Why? It saves you from the interrogation that will follow. A good number of people simply don't understand the plant-based lifestyle. Therefore, to avoid putting yourself in an awkward situation, simply serve your ideal veg-friendly diet and eat.

Trouble Locating Restaurants

Locating restaurants that offer plant-based diets is another major problem that vegans and vegetarians have to go through. Fortunately, from what we discussed earlier on, you can take advantage of the convenience that apps bring to us. Mobile applications can make it easy for you to locate restaurants based on the dishes they serve. Thus, with a few taps on your phone, you can easily find where you can enjoy time with friends and family.

Transitioning Pains and Woes

Of course, there are side effects that you will experience during the early stages of your transformation. Any change in diet can certainly spur a series of complications. Your metabolic process is going through a drastic change. Hence, you should expect symptoms such as bloating and gas. Your body will be adapting to a diet rich in fiber, so expect these changes to affect you.

The Possibility of Higher Cost

We discussed how you can stick to your plant-based diet while running on a budget. Many people end up giving up on the idea of going vegan because of the assumed expenses. However, this is not always the case. A well-planned diet plan should make it easy for you to maintain a healthy diet while following your budget.

Health Uncertainty

There are many changes that you will be making, not only to your diet plan, but also to your general lifestyle. Honestly, this will not be an easy move. You will be hesitant about the changes that you will be making. This is the dilemma that most of us have to go through when we are forced to try different diets with the hopes of improving our health or losing weight. As a result, many questions will come to your mind concerning plant-based diets and whether or not the change will help you meet the goals you have in mind. This is a challenge that you have to overcome through experimentation and research.

You will have to continue trying different diets until you find one that suits you. Moreover, research will help you achieve an in-depth understanding that there is a lot to gain from sticking to plant-based foods.

When you consider the challenges that you will face when changing your diet, you should be motivated knowing that these challenges are simply avoided. There are many health benefits that you will gain by choosing plant foods. As such, it is worth the risk to face these challenges and live a healthier and happier life.

Tips for Nutritional Goals

Nutritional Goals

As you set out on your nutritional path to changing your diet and hoping to get the best from it, you will have to set goals. When doing this, it is essential that you set smart goals. This means that the goals you set should be specific, measurable, actionable, realistic, and time-bound. Hence, your goals should help you reach your potential and benefit from the plant-based diet that you will be choosing. The significance of setting these goals is that they will help in reminding you of the bigger picture in spite of the challenges that you will face. Regardless of how many times you might fail, your goals will keep you motivated.

Setting Health Goals

Perhaps the primary reason why you might choose to turn to a plant-based lifestyle is to lose weight. Alternatively, it could be that you are looking to reverse diabetes that you have just been diagnosed with. Whatever reason you have, you should create goals that are centered around your overall health. Therefore, don't limit your goals to your weight loss plan. Set goals to improve your general health, as this will motivate you with the weekly strides you will be making.

Kitchen Goals

Since you are turning to a plant-based diet, this means that you will be spending more time cooking. Working in a clean and organized environment will help you stick to your diet plan. Why? It will help you enjoy spending time in the kitchen and learning how to cook new dishes. Setting your kitchen goals also implies that you should shop for new items, including cooking utensils, and fill your fridge with the right foods. The makeover to a new diet plan should be evident right from your kitchen. So, ensure that you give it the best look.

Setting Goals for Fruit and Vegetable Intake

With your new plant-based diet plan, you will experience a major change in the number of fruits and veggies you will be consuming. To help you stay on track, you should set daily intake goals. For instance, set a goal to eat two or three fruits in a day. At the same time, there are certain vegetables that should be part of your daily intake goal. Meeting these goals assures you that you are on the right path towards being healthy. Moreover, you will maintain your motivation that your ultimate goal of enjoying a healthy life is possible and attainable.

Protein Goals

A lot has been said about the concerns of plant-based diets being incomplete. We have come to the conclusion that, despite the ability to get all the nutrients from plant-based foods, it is still important to fill in the gaps with recommended supplements. In relation to this issue, you should take the time to set daily protein goals. You don't want to deprive your body of any vital nutrient. Consequently, setting goals for your daily protein intake is fundamental.

Eating at Home Goals

There are a few tips we previously discussed about dining at restaurants. Without a doubt, eating out is enjoyable. You get to have fun with friends and family. Nevertheless, it will be a huge challenge when you change your diet. For that reason, you should set clear goals to try your best to limit your eating in restaurants. For instance, you can set the objective of eating at home for five days. This is a great way of making sure that you maintain your diet. You should also understand that eating at home warrants that you indulge in clean eating most of the time. Create a timetable that will help you develop a habit of eating at home. Ultimately, you will enjoy the benefits that come with it.

New Recipe Goals

The last thing that you want as you try and transition to plant-based diets is boring meals. This will only discourage you and you might end up submitting to your cravings for animal foods. You should make an effort to try new recipes daily, weekly, or monthly depending on your schedule. Trying out different types of plant-based recipes will help bring some excitement to your diet plan. Your curiosity will assist you in developing a positive outlook on what you are trying to do.

The best thing about trying out new recipes is that you will gradually enhance your cooking skills. You will find remarkable ways of adding a new flavor to your dishes to keep you interested. In time, you shouldn't be surprised that your family and friends will want to join you in eating plant-based foods.

Keep a Journal

Your new vegan or vegetarian lifestyle will take different turns from time to time. Some days you will enjoy the smooth transition, and on other days you will feel discouraged. Well, this is normal. A great way to ensure that you remember all these moments is by keeping a journal. This journal should state your daily, weekly, or monthly goals and whether you managed to achieve them. Take note of the fact that your journal could help you determine your favorite dishes from the plant-based catalog you will have. Therefore, in addition to tracking your progress, keeping a journal will help keep you focused on your daily and weekly goals.

Evidently, setting nutritional goals as you move from animal-based foods to plant-based foods is key to making your health dreams a reality. If you have struggled to meet your health goals, then you will definitely understand why and how this is important. Nothing should be taken for granted. Whether you are organizing your kitchen or preparing a plant-only shopping list, everything should be planned for. Setting clear goals concerning what you want to achieve by eating plant foods is vital. This way, you don't approach the entire process blindly without knowing what to expect.

Chapter 4: The Food Lover's Plant-Based Kitchen

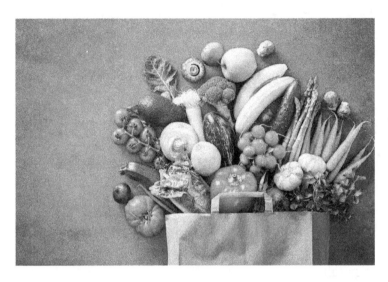

To succeed and make yourself accountable, you have to shape your environment to match your goals—starting with what you bring into your kitchen and put into your body. If you make sure you have a variety of healthy foods in your kitchen, you can always pull together a balanced meal. Even if you don't have exactly what a specific recipe calls for, you should have the components you need for substitutions. Let's give your kitchen a makeover.

The Pantry

Let's toss the refined flours, sugars, and oils, and opt instead for wholesome, unrefined versions. Stock up on whole grains, beans and legumes, and dried fruit.

83

- Whole grains (brown rice, quinoa, buckwheat, millet)

- Beans and legumes (chickpeas, kidney beans, lentils)

- Dried fruit (raisins, dates, dried apricots, cranberries)

- Unrefined oils (olive, coconut, toasted sesame)

- Vinegar (apple cider, balsamic, wine)

- Whole-grain flours (whole wheat, spelt, oat, buckwheat)

- Unrefined sweeteners (whole unrefined cane sugar like sucanat, coconut sugar, maple syrup, molasses, pure stevia)

- Sea salt

- Spices (ginger, cumin, coriander, turmeric, paprika, cinnamon)

- Dried herbs (basil, oregano, thyme, dill, herb mixes)

- Nutritional yeast

The Refrigerator

- Let's toss the meats, cheeses, milk, eggs, and packaged meals. Stock up on fresh produce, nuts and seeds, and non-dairy choices.

- Leafy greens (lettuce, kale, chard, spinach)

84

- Fresh herbs and spices (parsley, basil, mint, garlic, ginger)

- Green/non-starchy vegetables (cucumber, bell peppers, green beans, broccoli, mushrooms)

- Starchy vegetables (carrots, beets, sweet potato, winter squash)

- Onions (sweet, red, yellow, green)

- Fruit (apples, oranges, plums, grapes, melon)

- Nuts and seeds (almonds, pecans, sunflower seeds, chia seeds, flaxseed)

- Nut and seed butter (peanut, almond, cashew, sunflower)

- Non-dairy milk (almond, soy)

The Freezer

Time to ditch the TV dinners, French fries, frozen waffles, ice cream, frozen pies, and cakes. Stock up on fresh-frozen produce and homemade stuff.

- Frozen berries, mango, melon

- Frozen ripe bananas for smoothies and creamy sorbet

- Frozen edamame beans, peas, corn, broccoli, spinach, and other fresh-frozen whole vegetables

85

- The food you cook in big batches and freeze in single servings (soups, stews, chili, tomato sauce, veggie burgers)

- Healthy desserts (whole-food brownies, muffins, cookies, fruit pies)

Cooking Equipment

Healthy eating doesn't require any special equipment, but there are some things I use regularly and think you will be glad to have on hand when you make my recipes. However, there are ways to get around most things, so I'll tell you what you really need, and what would just be nice to have.

Essential Items

Good knives. No way around this one. One of the absolute best kitchen tools you can have is a good knife. They make such a huge difference in the speed and control you have in food prep. I'm always reminded of that when I travel and have to use cheap and/or dull knives. If you're short on cash, just buy one good chef's knife and one paring knife. They'll cover most jobs, and are much more useful than a full set of cheap knives.

Cutting board. Wood or bamboo are best to prolong the life of your knife. Flavors get trapped in them, so you may get a hint of garlic or onion with your mango, unless you have two cutting boards. Plastic (bonus if it's recycled) is a good way to minimize flavor combinations but doesn't offer much protection for your knife, so layer plastic on top of wood or bamboo for the best of both worlds. The bigger the surface area, the better.

Pots and pans. Just a few good ones will do: one big soup pot and one smaller pot for cooking rice, both with lids, and one big sauté pan or skillet. You'll also need a baking sheet, a pie pan, and an eight-inch or nine-inch square baking pan. I like stainless steel or tempered glass for pots, stainless steel or cast iron for skillets, and glass for baking dishes. Ceramic coatings are a good nonstick option for skillets.

Measuring cups and spoons. Get a stainless steel or ceramic set rather than plastic.

Cooking utensils. There are lots of little things, like a stirring spoon, ladle, flipper and spatula that you'll find you need in the course of your budding kitchen adventures.

Immersion or hand blender. This is the best way to purée soup and mashed potatoes. You can use a blender or food processor if you have one, or simply eat soups loose instead of puréed. You could even get away with a potato masher if you're okay with a chunky soup.

Blender and/or food processor. Use a blender to make smoothies, soups, and sauces. You don't need to spend $400; the $20 blenders are perfectly adequate for most functions. Food processors are much more versatile, so if you can only have one appliance, I'd suggest a food processor. They do tend to cost more than blenders, though. If you need a low-cost option, try a thrift store; they often have used food processors fairly cheap.

Garlic press. A garlic press pulverizes garlic cloves, which will meld the garlic flavor more smoothly into your dishes. Crushing also activates the antioxidants in garlic.

Citrus zester. A zester takes the very outside of a citrus peel, which contains a huge amount of flavor and antioxidants. Once you start adding orange, lemon, and lime zest to your cooking, you won't be able to look at a citrus fruit without thinking of what you can put that zest into. Many people also use Microplanes (very fine graters) instead of a zester. I love the visual of the thin curls that come from my zester, and I bought it for a dollar at a thrift store, so I stick with that. But if you already have a grater for zesting, there's probably no need to get another tool for the same purpose.

Ginger grater. This enables you to grate a piece, and squeeze the juice from it. It gives your meal a nice ginger kick, but in a smooth and even way. You can do this with a normal grater or a Microplane, but a ginger grater does a better job of ripping the ginger into a pulp and keeping it all together so that you get more of the juice.

Sprouting jars. Sprouts (like alfalfa or clover) are full of nutrients, and making your own at home offers maximum nutrition. You can use mason jars topped with mesh held on with an elastic band for sprouting, but the sprouts made in a sprouting jar are usually better quality because they have better drainage and airflow. They also make it a lot easier to rinse the sprouts, so I'm more likely to do it when I'm supposed to. If you compare the jar to the cost of buying sprouts from the grocery store, it's well worth it.

Oil sprayer. Not the aerosols but the kind you fill up with your own choice of oil and then pump to build up pressure and spray. They're fantastic for getting a fine mist of oil on veggies (rather than drizzling too much) for roasting, or seasoning your cast iron pan.

How to Purify Your Kitchen and Your Shopping

When you have a system in place, it is not difficult to plan your meals. There are, however, a few things you will need to keep in mind when you start. These tips will help you make the process of meal planning easier for you.

Have A Template

Don't start from scratch every week. Instead, create a template and list the type of food that you want to cook on each day of the week. You should also make note of the number of times you want to use the main ingredient during the week, so you can buy it accordingly.

Focus on Core Recipes

When you find the recipes that your family enjoys, make those dishes your core recipes. Try and identify those recipes and use them whenever you can. Ensure that you identify at least twenty as core recipes, and use at least five such recipes every week. You can try the different options in this book to find the lunch and dinner recipes that your family prefers. You can even refer to the previous book and identify core plant-based breakfast recipes.

Consume Leftovers for Breakfast and Lunch

It is hard to break out of the habit of consuming bread or a bowl of cereal every morning for breakfast. There is, however, an easy way to consume healthy food for breakfast if you plan your meals. All you need to do is prepare extra portions of your meals and jazz them up a bit and serve for breakfast. Keep an eye on the dishes that your kids love and serve them for breakfast. You will be surprised how easily they finish their breakfast! If stored properly, these recipes also become a good substitute for untimely snacks.

Now that you are aware of meal planning, let us look at some recipes that you can use to plan your meals in advance. The best part about these recipes is they are all cooked using healthy ingredients, so you don't have to worry about providing your family with the best nutrition; I've got you covered. All these recipes are easy to make and high on nutrition. You can even substitute certain ingredients with other ingredients of your choice and add a personal twist to the recipe.

Chapter 5: Plant-Based Breakfast

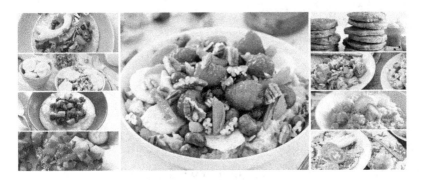

Commended Foods and Dishes

There are several options that can be eaten under a plant-based diet. They include the following:

- Granola

- Breakfast cereal

- Oatmeal

- Bananas

- Mangoes

- Tofu

- Mushrooms

- Cereals

- Oranges

- Berries

- Dates

There are a whole lot of plant-based foods that are available to be eaten. Make your choice according to what you prefer.

The Importance of a Good Breakfast

Cognitive Function

Breakfast is important in the restoration of essential carbs and glucose levels needed for the proper function of the brain. Breakfast provides energy and also improves the levels of concentration and memory thereby making us happier than we are because it lowers the levels of stress.

Breakfast has been found to improve behavior, attainment and attainment and improved grades.

Energy Needs

A good breakfast provides you with energy that will enable you to jumpstart your day. The levels of energy needed vary from one person to another depending on age, sex, etc.

Alternative Milk, Alternative Egg, Alternative Cheese

Some of the plant-based milk alternatives include;

- Coconut milk

- Hazelnut milk.

- Macadamia milk.

- Cashew milk.

- Oat milk.

- Almond milk.

Plant-based egg alternatives include algae and soy protein. Instead of using dairy cheese, you can make plant-based cheese made of seasonings, nutritional yeast and cashews.

Examples and Recipes of Well-Balanced Plant-Based Breakfasts

Homemade Granola

Prep time: 5 minutes

Cook time: 1 hour 15 minutes

Serves: 7

Ingredients:

- 5 cups rolled oats
- 1 cup almonds, slivered
- ¾ cup coconut, shredded
- ¾ tsp salt
- ¼ cup coconut oil
- ½ cup maple syrup

Instructions:

1. Preheat oven to 250°F.
2. Mix all ingredients in a large bowl.
3. Spread granola evenly on two rimmed sheet pans.
4. Bake at 250°F for 1 hour 15 minutes, stirring every 20-25 min.
5. Let cool in pans, and serve.

Nutritional Value Per Serving:

Calories 239; Fats 11 g; Carbohydrates 32 g; Protein 6 g

Country Breakfast Cereal

Prep time: 5 minutes

Cook time: 40 minutes

Serves: 6

Ingredients:

- 1 cup brown rice, uncooked
- ½ cup raisins, seedless
- 1 tsp cinnamon, ground
- ¼ Tbsp butter
- 2 ¼ cups water
- Honey, to taste
- Nuts, toasted

Instructions:

1. Combine rice, butter, raisins, and cinnamon in a saucepan. Add 2 ¼ cups water. Bring to boil.

2. Simmer covered for 40 minutes until rice is tender.

3. Fluff with fork. Add honey and nuts to taste.

Nutritional Value Per Serving:

Calories 160; Carbohydrates 34 g; Fats 1.5 g; Protein 3 g

Oatmeal Fruit Shake

Prep time: 10 minutes

Cook time: 0 minutes

Serves: 2

Ingredients:

- 1 cup oatmeal, already prepared, cooled
- 1 apple, cored, roughly chopped
- 1 banana, halved
- 1 cup baby spinach
- 2 cups coconut water
- 2 cups ice, cubed
- ½ tsp ground cinnamon
- 1 tsp pure vanilla extract

Instructions:

1. Add all ingredients to a blender.
2. Blend from low to high for several minutes until smooth.

Nutritional Value Per Serving:

Calories 270

Carbohydrates 58 g

Fats 1.5 g

Protein 5 g

Amaranth Banana Breakfast Porridge

Prep time: 10 minutes

Cook time: 25 minutes

Serves: 8

Ingredients:

- 2 cup amaranth

- 2 cinnamon sticks

- 4 bananas, diced

- 2 Tbsp chopped pecans

- 4 cups water

Instructions:

1. Combine the amaranth, water, and cinnamon sticks, and banana in a pot. Cover and let simmer around 25 minutes.

2. Remove from heat and discard the cinnamon. Places into bowls, and top with pecans.

Nutritional Value Per Serving:

Calories 330

Carbohydrates 62 g

Fats 6 g

Protein 10 g

Breakfast Quinoa with Figs and Honey

Prep time: 5 minutes

Cook time: 15 minutes

Serves: 4

Ingredients:

- 2 cups water
- 1 cup white quinoa
- 1 cup dried figs, sliced
- 1 cup walnuts, chopped
- 1 cup almond milk
- ½ tsp cinnamon, ground
- ¼ tsp cloves, ground
- Honey, to taste

Instructions:

1. Rinse quinoa under cool water.
2. Combine it with water, cinnamon, and cloves. Bring to boil.
3. Simmer covered for 10-15 minutes.
4. Add dried figs, nuts, milk. Garnish with honey. Serve.

Nutritional Value Per Serving:

Calories 420; Carbohydrates 55 g; Fats 20 g; Protein 11 g

Maple Walnut Teff Porridge

Prep time: 5 minutes

Cook time: 20 minutes

Serves: 2

Ingredients:

- 1 ½ cups water
- 1 cup teff, whole grain
- ½ cup coconut milk
- ½ tsp cardamom, ground
- ¼ cup walnuts, chopped
- 1 tsp sea salt
- 1 Tbsp maple syrup

Instructions:

1. Combine the water and coconut oil in a medium pot. Bring to boil, then stir in the teff.

2. Add the cardamom, and simmer uncovered for 15-20 minutes.

3. Mix in the maple syrup and walnuts. Serve.

Nutritional Value Per Serving:

Calories 312; Carbohydrates 35 g; Fats 18 g; Protein 7 g

PB & J Overnight Oatmeal

Prep time: 25 minutes

Cook time: 8 hours 20 minutes

Serves: 4

Ingredients:

- 1½ cups blueberries, frozen
- 4 Tbsp chia seeds, divided
- 2 cups rolled oats
- 3 cups almond milk
- 4 pitted dates
- 2 Tbsp peanut butter

Instructions:

1. Microwave blueberries in 1 Tbsp water for 2-3 minutes.
2. Stir in 2 Tbsp chia seed to the blueberries. Refrigerate for 20 minutes.
3. Put ½ cup oats and ½ Tbsp chia seeds into 4 jars.
4. Blend milk, dates, and peanut butter. Pour it into the jars.
5. Add blueberry chia jam to the jars. Refrigerate for 6-8 hours.

Nutritional Value Per Serving:

Calories 320; Carbohydrates 45 g; Fats 11 g; Protein 9 g

Southwest Tofu Scramble

Prep time: 10 minutes

Cook time: 15 minutes

Serves: 4

Ingredients:

- 1 package firm tofu, crumbled
- 1-2 tsp ground cumin
- ½ cup nutritional yeast
- 2 tsp tamari
- 2 tsp extra-virgin olive oil
- 1 zucchini, diced
- 1 bell pepper, diced
- 1 onion, diced

Instructions:

1. Mix the first four ingredients with a fork.
2. In a heavy skillet, combine the zucchini, pepper, shallot, and olive oil. Sauté for 5 minutes.
3. Stir in tofu and cook for another 10 minutes. Serve.

Nutritional Value Per Serving:

Calories 6.6 g; Carbohydrates 6.6 g; Fats 3.6 g; Protein 7 g

Amaranth Polenta with Wild Mushrooms

Prep time: 10 minutes

Cook time: 30 minutes

Serves: 3

Ingredients:

- ½ ounce dried porcini

- 1 Tbsp olive oil

- ¼ cup shallots, chopped

- 1 cup amaranth

- ¼ tsp salt

- 1 tsp fresh thyme, chopped

- Ground pepper, to taste

Instructions:

1. Combine 1 ¾ cups boiling water and mushrooms. Leave for 10 minutes to soften.

2. In a saucepan, cook shallots in olive oil for 1 minute. Add amaranth, mushrooms, and soaking liquid. Simmer for 15 minutes.

3. Add pepper, thyme, and salt. Simmer for another 15 minutes.

4. Serve in small bowls.

Nutritional Value Per Serving:

Calories 280; Carbohydrates 42 g; Fats 7 g; Protein 12 g

Berry Breakfast Bars

Prep time: 8 minutes; Cook time: 27 minutes; Serves: 9

Ingredients:

- 1 ½ cup Rolled oats
- ½ cup Applesauce
- 1 tablespoon Flaxseed meal
- 2 cups Almond flour
- ¼ Salt
- ¼ cup Blackstrap molasses
- ½ teaspoon Baking powder
- 1 teaspoon Vanilla extract
- ¼ cup Almond butter
- 1 teaspoon Apple cider vinegar
- ½ cup Oat milk
- ¼ cup Maple syrup
- 1 tablespoon Agar-agar
- 3 cups mixed frozen berries
- 1 teaspoon Lemon juice

Instructions:

1. You'll need an oven-safe dish, preferably a baking dish. Square is better to get nine full-portioned squares from it, but

105

any shape will do. Your oven should be heated to 350°F and your baking dish should be lined with baking paper.

2. Mix together the oat milk, applesauce, molasses, vanilla, and almond butter. Add the almond flour and flaxseed meal and mix. If it looks too thick at this point, add a little water (maybe a tablespoon or two) to ensure it is runny enough to accept the oats. Stir in the oats and baking powder then add the salt and mix really well to get a nice thick batter.

3. Spoon all but about one cup of mixture into the bottom of your dish and press it down with your fingers to get an even base and bake for 15 minutes.

4. While this is in the oven, get a saucepan and over medium-high heat, cook down the frozen berries and agar-agar with half a cup of cold water. Keep an eye on it and once it comes to a boil, you should turn down the heat to medium-low and let it simmer for around five minutes while stirring as it thickens. Then take it off the heat and add the lemon juice and maple syrup, stir again and then leave to thicken.

5. Pour this over the oat base and with your fingers, roughly crumble the cup of oat mixture you put aside over the top of the berry filling.

6. Put the baking dish back in the oven for another 12 minutes then take out. The oat mixture on top should be beautifully browned. Allow it to cool before you put it in the fridge to set for an hour or so.

7. Cut into squares or bars or whatever makes you happy. Then wrap individually in baking paper or cling film and keep in the fridge or freezer!

Nutritional Value Per Serving:

Calories 114; Carbohydrates 14 g; Fats 6 g; Protein 2 g

Chapter 6: Plant-Based Lunch

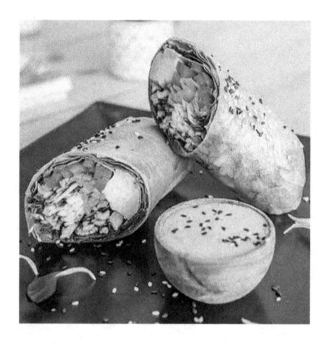

Commended Foods and Dishes

There are many options available for plant-based lunches. They include but not limited to the following;

- Vegetable salad

- Avocado

- Coconut

- Nuts

- Macadamia

- Vegetable salads

- Cereals

- Cashew nuts

- Zucchini sandwich

Foods to Avoid

The entire whole-food plant-based diet plan is based on adding natural food to your plate and avoiding as much artificially-produced food as possible. There is no space for heavily processed foods on a plant-based diet plan. This means that while you are purchasing grocery items, choose fresh foods. When you do buy packaged food, opt for the ones with the least amount of ingredients. Here are examples of foods you should avoid:

- Pork

- Game Meats

- Sheep

- Beef

- Eggs

- Dairy

- Poultry

- Seafood

Alternative Meat

- Impossible Burger

- Beyond Meat Burger

- Beyond Sausage.

- Lightlife Italian Sausage

- Abbot's Butcher "Chorizo"

- Nuggets

Examples and Recipes of Well-Balanced Plant-Based Meals

Cashew Siam Salad

Prep time: 10 minutes

Cook time: 3 minutes

Serves: 4

Ingredients:

Salad:

- 4 cups baby spinach, rinsed, drained
- ½ cup pickled red cabbage

Dressing:

- 1-inch piece ginger, finely chopped
- 1 tsp. chili garlic paste
- 1 tbsp. soy sauce
- ½ tbsp. rice vinegar
- 1 tbsp. sesame oil
- 3 tbsp. avocado oil

Toppings:

- ½ cup raw cashews, unsalted

- ¼ cup fresh cilantro, chopped

Instructions:

1. Put the spinach and red cabbage in a large bowl. Toss to combine and set the salad aside.

2. Toast the cashews in a frying pan over medium-high heat, stirring occasionally until the cashews are golden brown. This should take about 3 minutes. Turn off the heat and set the frying pan aside.

3. Mix all the dressing ingredients in a medium-sized bowl and use a spoon to mix them into a smooth dressing.

4. Pour the dressing over the spinach salad and top with the toasted cashews.

5. Toss the salad to combine all ingredients and transfer the large bowl to the fridge. Allow the salad to chill for up to one hour – doing so will guarantee a better flavor. Alternatively, the salad can be served right away, topped with the optional cilantro. Enjoy!

Nutritional Value Per Serving:

Calories 236

Carbohydrates 6.1 g

Fats 21.6 g

Protein 4.2 g

Avocado and Cauliflower Hummus

Prep time: 5 minutes

Cook time: 25 minutes

Serves: 2

Ingredients:

- 1 medium cauliflower, stem removed and chopped

- 1 large Hass avocado, peeled, pitted, and chopped

- ¼ cup extra virgin olive oil

- 2 garlic cloves

- ½ tbsp. lemon juice

- ½ tsp. onion powder

- Sea salt and ground black pepper to taste

- 2 large carrots

- ¼ cup fresh cilantro, chopped

Instructions:

1. Preheat the oven to 450°F, and line a baking tray with aluminum foil.

2. Put the chopped cauliflower on the baking tray and drizzle with 2 tablespoons of olive oil.

3. Roast the chopped cauliflower in the oven for 20-25 minutes, until lightly brown.

4. Remove the tray from the oven and allow the cauliflower to cool down.

5. Add all the ingredients—except the carrots and optional fresh cilantro—to a food processor or blender, and blend the ingredients into a smooth hummus.

6. Transfer the hummus to a medium-sized bowl, cover, and put it in the fridge for at least 30 minutes.

7. Take the hummus out of the fridge and, if desired, top it with the optional chopped cilantro and more salt and pepper to taste; serve with the carrot fries, and enjoy!

Nutritional Value Per Serving:

Calories 416

Carbohydrates 8.4 g

Fats 40.3 g

Protein 3.3 g

Raw Zoodles with Avocado 'N Nuts

Prep time: 10 minutes

Serves: 2

Ingredients:

- 1 medium zucchini
- 1½ cups basil
- 1/3 cup water
- 5 tbsp. pine nuts
- 2 tbsp. lemon juice
- 1 medium avocado, peeled, pitted, sliced
- Optional: 2 tbsp. olive oil
- 6 yellow cherry tomatoes, halved
- Optional: 6 red cherry tomatoes, halved
- Sea salt and black pepper to taste

Instructions:

1. Add the basil, water, nuts, lemon juice, avocado slices, optional olive oil (if desired), salt, and pepper to a blender.

2. Blend the ingredients into a smooth mixture. Add more salt and pepper to taste and blend again.

3. Divide the sauce and the zucchini noodles between two medium-sized bowls for serving, and combine in each.

4. Top the mixtures with the halved yellow cherry tomatoes, and the optional red cherry tomatoes (if desired); serve and enjoy!

Nutritional Value Per Serving:

Calories 317; Carbohydrates 7.4 g; Fats 28.1 g; Protein 7.2 g

Cauliflower Sushi

Prep time: 30 minutes

Serves: 4

Ingredients:

Sushi Base:

- 6 cups cauliflower florets

- ½ cup vegan cheese

- 1 medium spring onion, diced

- 4 nori sheets

- Sea salt and pepper to taste

- 1 tbsp. rice vinegar or sushi vinegar

- 1 medium garlic clove, minced

Filling:

- 1 medium Hass avocado, peeled, sliced

- ½ medium cucumber, skinned, sliced

- 4 asparagus spears

- A handful of enoki mushrooms

Instructions:

1. Put the cauliflower florets in a food processor or blender. Pulse the florets into a rice-like substance. When using readymade cauliflower rice, add this to the blender.

2. Add the vegan cheese, spring onions, and vinegar to the food processor or blender. Top these ingredients with salt and pepper to taste, and pulse everything into a chunky mixture. Make sure not to turn the ingredients into a puree by pulsing too long.

3. Taste and add more vinegar, salt, or pepper to taste. Add the optional minced garlic clove to the blender and pulse again for a few seconds.

4. Lay out the nori sheets and spread the cauliflower rice mixture out evenly between the sheets. Make sure to leave at least 2 inches of the top and bottom edges empty.

5. Place one or more combinations of multiple filling ingredients along the center of the spread out rice mixture. Experiment with different ingredients per nori sheet for the best flavor.

6. Roll up each nori sheet tightly. (Using a sushi mat will make this easier.)

7. Either serve the sushi as a nori roll, or, slice each roll up into sushi pieces.

8. Serve right away with a small amount of wasabi, pickled ginger, and soy sauce!

Nutritional Value Per Serving:

Calories 189; Carbohydrates 7.6 g; Fats 14.4 g; Protein 6.1 g

Spinach and Mashed Tofu Salad

Prep time: 20 minutes

Serves: 4

Ingredients:

- 2 8-oz. blocks firm tofu, drained
- 4 cups baby spinach leaves
- 4 tbsp. cashew butter
- 1½ tbsp. soy sauce
- 1-inch piece ginger, finely chopped
- 1 tsp. red miso paste
- 2 tbsp. sesame seeds
- 1 tsp. organic orange zest
- 1 tsp. nori flakes
- 2 tbsp. water

Instructions:

1. Use paper towels to absorb any excess water left in the tofu before crumbling both blocks into small pieces.

2. In a large bowl, combine the mashed tofu with the spinach leaves.

3. Mix the remaining ingredients in another small bowl and, if desired, add the optional water for a more smooth dressing.

4. Pour this dressing over the mashed tofu and spinach leaves.

5. Transfer the bowl to the fridge and allow the salad to chill for up to one hour. Doing so will guarantee a better flavor. Or, the salad can be served right away. Enjoy!

Nutritional Value Per Serving:

Calories 166

Carbohydrates 5.5 g

Fats 10.7 g

Protein 11.3 g

Cucumber Edamame Salad

Prep time: 5 minutes

Cook time: 8 minutes

Serves: 2

Ingredients:

- 3 tbsp. avocado oil
- 1 cup cucumber, sliced into thin rounds
- ½ cup fresh sugar snap peas, sliced or whole
- ½ cup fresh edamame
- ¼ cup radish, sliced
- 1 large Hass avocado, peeled, pitted, sliced
- 1 nori sheet, crumbled
- 2 tsp. roasted sesame seeds
- 1 tsp. salt

Instructions:

1. Bring a medium-sized pot filled halfway with water to a boil over medium-high heat.

2. Add the sugar snaps and cook them for about 2 minutes.

3. Take the pot off the heat, drain the excess water, transfer the sugar snaps to a medium-sized bowl and set aside for now.

4. Fill the pot with water again, add the teaspoon of salt and bring to a boil over medium-high heat.

5. Add the edamame to the pot and let them cook for about 6 minutes.

6. Take the pot off the heat, drain the excess water, transfer the soybeans to the bowl with sugar snaps and let them cool down for about 5 minutes.

7. Combine all ingredients, except the nori crumbs and roasted sesame seeds, in a medium-sized bowl.

8. Carefully stir, using a spoon, until all ingredients are evenly coated in oil.

9. Top the salad with the nori crumbs and roasted sesame seeds.

10. Transfer the bowl to the fridge and allow the salad to cool for at least 30 minutes.

11. Serve chilled and enjoy!

Nutritional Value Per Serving:

Calories 409

Carbohydrates 7.1 g

Fats 38.25 g

Protein 7.6 g

Artichoke White Bean Sandwich Spread

Prep time: 10 minutes

Serves: 2

Ingredients:

- ½ cup raw cashews, chopped
- Water
- 1 clove garlic, cut into half
- 1 tablespoon lemon zest
- 1 teaspoon fresh rosemary, chopped
- ¼ teaspoon salt
- ¼ teaspoon pepper
- 6 tablespoons almond, soy or coconut milk
- 1 15.5-ounce can cannellini beans, rinsed and drained well
- 3 to 4 canned artichoke hearts, chopped
- ¼ cup hulled sunflower seeds
- Green onions, chopped, for garnish

Instructions:

1. Soak the raw cashews for 15 minutes in enough water to cover them. Drain and dab with a paper towel to make them as dry as possible.

2. Transfer the cashews to a blender and add the garlic, lemon zest, rosemary, salt and pepper. Pulse to break everything up and then add the milk, one tablespoon at a time, until the mixture is smooth and creamy.

3. Mash the beans in a bowl with a fork. Add the artichoke hearts and sunflower seeds. Toss to mix.

4. Pour the cashew mixture on top and season with more salt and pepper if desired. Mix the ingredients well and spread on whole-wheat bread, crackers, or a wrap.

Nutritional Value Per Serving:

Calories 110

Carbohydrates 14 g

Fats 4 g

Protein 6 g

Buffalo Chickpea Wraps

Prep time: 20 minutes

Cook time: 5 minutes

Serves: 4

Ingredients:

- ¼ cup plus 2 tablespoons hummus
- 2 tablespoons lemon juice
- 1½ tablespoons maple syrup
- 1 to 2 tablespoons hot water
- 1 head Romaine lettuce, chopped
- 1 15-ounce can chickpeas, drained, rinsed and patted dry
- 4 tablespoons hot sauce, divided
- 1 tablespoon olive or coconut oil
- ¼ teaspoon garlic powder
- 1 pinch sea salt
- 4 wheat tortillas
- ¼ cup cherry tomatoes, diced
- ¼ cup red onion, diced
- ¼ of a ripe avocado, thinly sliced

Instructions:

1. Mix the hummus with the lemon juice and maple syrup in a large bowl. Use a whisk and add the hot water, a little at a time until it is thick but spreadable.

2. Add the Romaine lettuce and toss to coat. Set aside.

3. Pour the prepared chickpeas into another bowl. Add three tablespoons of the hot sauce, the olive oil, garlic powder and salt; toss to coat.

4. Heat a metal skillet (cast iron works the best) over medium heat and add the chickpea mixture. Sauté for three to five minutes and mash gently with a spoon.

5. Once the chickpea mixture is slightly dried out, remove from the heat and add the rest of the hot sauce. Stir it in well and set aside.

6. Lay the tortillas on a clean, flat surface and spread a quarter cup of the buffalo chickpeas on top. Top with tomatoes, onion and avocado (optional) and wrap.

Nutritional Value Per Serving:

Calories 254

Carbohydrates 39.4 g

Fats 6.7 g

Protein 9.1 g

Coconut Veggie Wraps

Prep time: 5 minutes

Serves: 5

Ingredients:

- 1½ cups shredded carrots

- 1 red bell pepper, seeded, thinly sliced

- 2½ cups kale

- 1 ripe avocado, thinly sliced

- 1 cup fresh cilantro, chopped

- 5 coconut wraps

- 2/3 cups hummus

- 6½ cups green curry paste

Instructions:

1. Slice, chop and shred all the vegetables.

2. Lay a coconut wrap on a clean flat surface and spread two tablespoons of the hummus and one tablespoon of the green curry paste on top of the end closest to you.

3. Place some carrots, bell pepper, kale and cilantro on the wrap and start rolling it up, starting from the edge closest to you. Roll tightly and fold in the ends.

4. Place the wrap, seam down, on a plate to serve.

Nutritional Value Per Serving:

Calories 236; Carbohydrates 23.6 g; Fats 14.3 g; Protein 5.5 g

Cucumber Avocado Sandwich

Prep time: 15 minutes

Serves: 2

Ingredients:

- ½ of a large cucumber, peeled, sliced

- ¼ teaspoon salt

- 4 slices whole-wheat bread

- 4 ounces goat cheese with or without herbs, at room temperature

- 2 Romaine lettuce leaves

- 1 large avocado, peeled, pitted, sliced

- 2 pinches lemon pepper

- 1 squeeze of lemon juice

- ½ cup alfalfa sprouts

Instructions:

1. Peel and slice the cucumber thinly. Lay the slices on a plate and sprinkle them with a quarter to a half teaspoon of salt. Let this set for 10 minutes or until water appears on the plate.

2. Place the cucumber slices in a colander and rinse with cold water. Let these drain, then place them on a dry plate and pat dry with a paper towel.

3. Spread all slices with goat cheese and place lettuce leaves on the two bottom pieces of bread.

4. Layer the cucumber slices and avocado atop the bread.

5. Sprinkle one pinch of lemon pepper over each sandwich and drizzle a little lemon juice over the top.

6. Top with the alfalfa sprouts and place another piece of bread, goat cheese down, on top.

Nutritional Value Per Serving:

Calories 246

Carbohydrates 20 g

Fats 12 g

Protein 9 g

Lentil Sandwich Spread

Prep time: 15 minutes

Cook time: 20 minutes

Serves: 3

Ingredients:

- 1 tablespoon water or oil
- 1 small onion, chopped
- 2 cloves garlic, minced
- 1 cup dry lentils
- 2 cups vegetable stock
- 1 tablespoon apple cider vinegar
- 2 tablespoons tomato paste
- 3 sun-dried tomatoes
- 2 tablespoons maple
- 1 teaspoon dried oregano
- ½ teaspoon ground cumin
- 1 teaspoon coriander
- 1 teaspoon turmeric
- ½ lemon, juiced

- 1 tablespoon fresh parsley, chopped

Instructions:

1. Warm a Dutch oven over medium heat and add the water or oil.

2. Immediately add the onions and sauté for two to three minutes or until softened. Add more water if this starts to stick to the pan.

3. Add the garlic and sauté for one minute.

4. Add the lentils, vegetable stock and vinegar; bring to a boil. Turn down to a simmer and cook for 15 minutes or until the lentils are soft and the liquid is almost completely absorbed.

5. Ladle the lentils into a food processor and add the tomato paste, sun-dried tomatoes and syrup; process until smooth.

6. Add the oregano, cumin, coriander, turmeric and lemon; processes until thoroughly mixed.

7. Remove the spread to a bowl and apply it to bread, toast, a wrap, or pita. Sprinkle With toppings as desired.

Nutritional Value Per Serving:

Calories 360

Carbohydrates 60.7 g

Fats 5.4 g

Protein 17.5 g

Mediterranean Tortilla Pinwheels

Prep time: 5 minutes

Cook time: 1 minute

Serves: 16

Ingredients:

- ½ cup water
- 4 tablespoons white vinegar
- 3 tablespoons lemon juice
- 3 tablespoons tahini paste
- 1 clove garlic, minced
- Salt and pepper to taste
- Canned artichokes, drained, thinly sliced
- Cherry tomatoes, thinly sliced
- Olives, thinly sliced
- Lettuce or baby spinach
- Tortillas

Instructions:

1. In a bowl, combine the water, vinegar, lemon juice and Tahini paste; whisk together until smooth.

2. Add the garlic, salt and pepper to taste; whisk to combine. Set the bowl aside.

3. Lay a tortilla on a flat surface and spread with one tablespoon of the sauce.

4. Lay some lettuce or spinach slices on top, then scatter some artichoke, tomato and olive slices on top.

5. Tightly roll the tortilla and fold in the sides. Cut the ends off and then slice into four or five pinwheels.

Nutritional Value Per Serving:

Calories 322

Carbohydrates 5 g

Fats 4 g

Protein 30 g

Rice and Bean Burritos

Prep time: 10 minutes

Cook time: 15 minutes

Serves: 8

Ingredients:

- 2 16-ounce cans fat-free refried beans

- 6 tortillas

- 2 cups cooked rice

- ½ cup salsa

- 1 tablespoon olive oil

- 1 bunch green onions, chopped

- 2 bell peppers, finely chopped

- Guacamole

Instructions:

1. Preheat the oven to 375°F.

2. Dump the refried beans into a saucepan and place over medium heat to warm.

3. Heat the tortillas and lay them out on a flat surface.

4. Spoon the beans in a long mound that runs across the tortilla, just a little off from center.

5. Spoon some rice and salsa over the beans; add the green pepper and onions to taste, along with any other finely chopped vegetables you like.

6. Fold over the shortest edge of the plain tortilla and roll it up, folding in the sides as you go.

7. Place each burrito, seam side down, on a nonstick-sprayed baking sheet.

8. Brush with olive oil and bake for 15 minutes.

9. Serve with guacamole.

Nutritional Value Per Serving:

Calories 290; Carbohydrates 49 g; Fats 6 g; Protein 9 g

Ricotta Basil Pinwheels

Prep: 10 minutes

Serves 4

Ingredients:

- ½ cup unsalted cashews

- Water

- 7 ounces firm tofu, cut into pieces

- ¼ cup almond milk

- 1 teaspoon white wine vinegar

- 1 clove garlic, smashed

- 20 to 25 fresh basil leaves

- Salt and pepper to taste

- 8 tortillas

- 7 ounces fresh spinach

- ½ cup black olives, sliced

- 2 to 3 tomatoes, cut into small pieces

Instructions:

1. Soak the cashews for 30 minutes in enough water to cover them. Drain them well and pat them dry with paper towels.

2. Place the cashews in a blender along with the tofu, almond milk, vinegar, garlic, basil leaves, salt and pepper to taste. Blend until smooth and creamy.

3. Spread the resulting mixture on the eight tortillas, dividing it equally.

4. Top with spinach leaves, olives and tomatoes.

5. Tightly roll each loaded tortilla.

6. Cut off the ends with a sharp knife and slice into four or five pinwheels.

Delicious Sloppy Joes With No Meat

Prep time: 6 minutes

Cook time: 5 minutes

Serves: 4

Ingredients:

- 5 tablespoons vegetable stock
- 2 stalks celery, diced
- 1 small onion, diced
- 1 small red bell pepper, diced
- 1 teaspoon garlic powder
- 1 teaspoon chili powder
- 1 teaspoon ground cumin

- 1 teaspoon salt

- 1 cup cooked bulgur wheat

- 1 cup red lentils

- 1 15-ounce can tomato sauce

- 4 tablespoons tomato paste

- 3½ cups water

- 2 teaspoons balsamic vinegar

- 1 tablespoon Hoisin sauce

Instructions:

1. In a Dutch oven, heat up the vegetable stock and add the celery, onion and bell pepper. Sauté until vegetables are soft, about five minutes.

2. Add the garlic powder, chili powder, cumin and salt and mix in.

3. Add the bulgur wheat, lentils, tomato sauce, tomato paste, water, vinegar and Hoisin sauce. Stir and bring to a boil.

4. Turn the heat down to a simmer and cook uncovered for 30 minutes. Stir occasionally to prevent sticking and scorching.

5. Taste to see if the lentils are tender.

6. When the lentils are done, serve on buns.

Nutritional Value Per Serving:

Calories 451; Fats 10 g; Carbohydrates 61 g; Protein 27 g

Spicy Hummus and Apple Wrap

Prep time: 10 minutes

Serves: 1

Ingredients:

- 3 to 4 tablespoons hummus

- 2 tablespoons mild salsa

- ½ cup broccoli slaw

- ½ teaspoon fresh lemon juice

- 2 teaspoons plain yogurt

- salt and pepper to taste

- 1 tortilla

- Lettuce leaves

- ½ Granny Smith or another tart apple, cored and thinly sliced

Instructions:

1. In a small bowl, mix the hummus with the salsa. Set the bowl aside.

2. In a large bowl, mix the broccoli slaw, lemon juice and yogurt. Season with the salt and pepper.

3. Lay the tortilla on a flat surface and spread on the hummus mixture.

137

4. Lay down some lettuce leaves on top of the hummus.

5. On the upper half of the tortilla, place a pile of the broccoli slaw mixture and cover with the apples.

6. Fold and wrap.

Nutritional Value Per Serving:

Calories 121

Carbohydrates 27 g

Fats 2 g

Protein 4 g

Sun-dried Tomato Spread

Prep time: 20 minutes

Serves: 16

Ingredients:

- 1 cup sun-dried tomatoes

- 1 cup raw cashews

- Water for soaking tomatoes and cashews

- ½ cup water

- 1 clove garlic, minced

- 1 green onion, chopped

- 5 large basil leaves

- ½ teaspoon lemon juice

- ¼ teaspoon salt

- 1 dash pepper

- Hulled sunflower seeds

Instructions:

1. Soak tomatoes and cashews for 30 minutes in separate bowls, with enough water to cover them. Drain and pat dry.

2. Put the tomatoes and cashews in a food processor and puree them, drizzling the water in as it purees to make a smooth, creamy paste.

3. Add the garlic, onion, basil leaves, lemon juice, salt and pepper and mix thoroughly.

4. Scrape into a bowl, cover and refrigerate overnight.

5. Spread on bread or toast and sprinkle with sunflower seeds for a little added crunch.

Nutritional Value Per Serving:

Calories 60

Carbohydrates 5.6 g

Fats 4.2 g

Protein 1.2 g

Sweet Potato Sandwich Spread

Prep time: 10 minutes

Servings: 4

Ingredients:

- 1 large sweet potato baked, peeled
- 1 teaspoon cumin
- 1 teaspoon chili powder
- 1 teaspoon garlic powder
- Salt and pepper to taste
- 2 slices whole-wheat bread
- 1 to 2 tablespoons pinto beans, drained
- Lettuce

Instructions:

1. Bake and peel the sweet potato and mash it in a bowl. If it is too thick, add a little almond or coconut milk.

2. Mix in the cumin, chili powder, garlic powder, salt and pepper.

3. Spread the mixture on a slice of bread and spoon some beans on top.

4. Top with lettuce leaves and the other slice of bread.

Nutritional Value Per Serving:

Calories 253; Carbohydrates 49 g; Fats 6 g; Protein 8 g

Zucchini Sandwich with Balsamic Dressing

Prep time: 5 minutes

Cook time: 2 minutes

Serves: 2

Ingredients:

- 2 small zucchinis

- 1 tablespoon olive oil

- 4 cloves garlic, thinly sliced

- 1 tablespoon balsamic vinegar

- 1 large roasted red pepper, chopped

- 1 cup cannellini beans, rinsed, drained

- 2 whole-wheat sandwich rolls

- 6 to 8 basil leaves

- ½ teaspoon pepper

Instructions:

1. Add the oil to a hot skillet and sauté the garlic for one or two minutes or until it just starts to brown.

141

2. Add the zucchini strips and sauté in batches (don't overcrowd) and lay out on a plate until they are all finished.

3. Reduce heat to medium and place all the zucchini strips back in the pan.

4. Add the vinegar and sauté for about a minute.

5. In the blender, process the red pepper and beans until smooth.

6. Toast the buns and spoon onto the bottom halves the bean and pepper mixture.

7. Lay basil leaves on top and then the zucchini.

8. Grind some pepper on top and close the sandwich with the top of the bun.

Nutritional Value Per Serving:

Calories 274

Carbohydrates 50.1 g

Fats 2.5 g

Protein 16 g

Chapter 7: Plant-Based Dinner

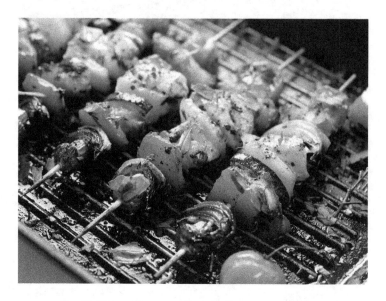

Commended Foods and Dishes

Some of the foods that you can eat are as follows:

- Chickpeas

- Black beans

- White ice

- Herbs

- Brown rice

- Gigante beans

- Hummus

Alternative Pasta

- Black Bean Spaghetti

- Zucchini

- Shirataki Noodles

- Spaghetti Squash

Examples and Recipes of Well-Balanced Plant-Based Dinners

<u>Summer Harvest Pizza</u>

Prep time: 20 minutes

Cook time: 15 minutes

Serves: 2

Ingredients:

- 1 Lavash flatbread, whole grain

- 4 Tbsp Feta spread, store-bought

- ½ cup cheddar cheese, shredded

- ½ cup corn kernels, cooked

- ½ cup beans, cooked

- ½ cup fire-roasted red peppers, chopped

Instructions:

1. Preheat oven to 350°F.

2. Cut Lavash into two halves. Bake crusts on a pan in the oven for 5 minutes.

3. Spread feta spread on both crusts. Top with remaining ingredients.

4. Bake for another 10 minutes.

Nutritional Value Per Serving:

Calories 230

Carbohydrates 23 g

Fats 15 g

Protein 11 g

Whole Wheat Pizza with Summer Produce

Prep time: 15 minutes

Cook time: 15 minutes

Serves: 2

Ingredients:

- 1 pound whole wheat pizza dough
- 4 ounces goat cheese
- 2/3 cup blueberries
- 2 ears corn, husked
- 2 yellow squash, sliced
- 2 Tbsp olive oil

Instructions:

1. Preheat the oven to 450°F.
2. Roll the dough out to make a pizza crust.
3. Crumble the cheese on the crust. Spread remaining ingredients, then drizzle with olive oil.
4. Bake for about 15 minutes. Serve.

Nutritional Value Per Serving:

Calories 470; Carbohydrates 66 g; Fats 18 g; Protein 17 g

Spicy Chickpeas

Prep time: 15 minutes

Cook time: 20 minutes

Serves: 8

Ingredients:

- 1 Tbsp extra-virgin olive oil

- 1 yellow onion, diced

- 1 tsp curry

- ¼ tsp allspice

- 1 can diced tomatoes

- 2 cans chickpeas, rinsed, drained

- Salt, cayenne pepper, to taste

Instructions:

1. Simmer onions in 1 Tbsp oil for 4 minutes.

2. Add allspice and pepper, cook for 2 minutes.

3. Stir in tomatoes, and cook for another 2 minutes.

4. Add chickpeas, and simmer for 10 minutes.

5. Season with salt, and serve.

Nutritional Value Per Serving:

Calories 146; Carbohydrates 25 g; Fats 3 g; Protein 5 g

Farro with Pistachios & Herbs

Prep time: 20 minutes

Cook time: 45 minutes

Serves: 10

Ingredients:

- 2 cups farro

- 4 cups water

- 1 tsp kosher salt, divided

- 2½ Tbsp extra-virgin olive oil

- 1 onion, chopped

- 2 cloves garlic, minced

- ½ tsp ground pepper, divided

- ½ cup parsley, chopped

- 4 oz salted shelled pistachios, toasted, chopped

Instructions:

1. Combine farro, water, and ¾ tsp salt, simmer for 40 minutes.

2. Cook onion and garlic in 2 Tbsp oil for 5 minutes.

3. Combine ½ tsp oil, ¼ tsp pepper, parsley, pistachios, and toss well.

4. Combine all. Season with salt and pepper.

Nutritional Value Per Serving:

Calories 220; Carbohydrates 30 g; Fats 9 g; Protein 8 g

Millet and Teff with Squash & Onions

Prep time: 10 minutes

Cook time: 20 minutes

Serves: 6

Ingredients:

- 1 cup millet
- ½ cup teff grain
- 4½ cups of water
- 1 onion, sliced
- 1 butternut squash, chopped
- Sea salt, to taste

Instructions:

1. Rinse millet, and put in a large pot.
2. Add remaining ingredients. Mix well.
3. Simmer 20 minutes until all the water is absorbed.
4. Serve hot.

Nutritional Value Per Serving:

Calories 200; Carbohydrates 40 g; Fats 2 g; Protein 6 g

Brown Rice Tabbouleh

Prep time: 20 minutes

Cook time: 0 minutes

Serves: 6

Ingredients:

- 3 cups brown rice, cooked
- ¾ cup cucumber, chopped
- ¾ cup tomato, chopped
- ¼ cup mint leaves, chopped
- ¼ cup green onions, sliced
- ¼ cup olive oil
- ¼ cup lemon juice
- Salt, pepper, to taste

Instructions:

1. Combine all ingredients in a large bowl.
2. Toss well and chill for 20 min.

Nutritional Value Per Serving:

Calories 201; Carbohydrates 25 g; Fats 10 g; Protein 3 g

Healthy Hoppin' John

Prep time: 15 minutes

Cook time: 1 hour

Serves: 4

Ingredients:

- 1 Tbsp extra-virgin olive oil

- 1 onion, diced

- 2 garlic cloves, minced

- 1 cup of dried black-eyed peas

- 1 cup brown rice, uncooked

- 4 cups water

- Salt, pepper, to taste

Instructions:

1. Cook the onions and garlic in oil for 3 minutes.

2. Combine the peas, salt, brown rice, and 4 cups of water and bring to a boil.

3. Add pepper. Simmer for 45 minutes.

4. Serve hot.

Nutritional Value Per Serving:

Calories 248; Carbohydrates 47 g; Fats 5 g; Protein 6 g

Beans & Greens Bowl

Prep time: 2 minutes

Cook time: 2 minutes

Serves: 1

Ingredients:

- 1½ cups curly kale, washed, chopped

- ½ cup black beans, cooked

- ½ avocado

- 2 Tbsp feta cheese, crumbled

Instructions:

1. Mix the kale and black beans in a microwavable bowl and heat for about 1 ½ minute.

2. Add the avocado and stir well. Top with feta.

Nutritional Value Per Serving:

Calories 340

Carbohydrates 32 g

Fats 19 g

Protein 13 g

Black Beans & Brown Rice

Prep time: 2 minutes

Cook time: 45 minutes

Serves: 4

Ingredients:

- 4 cups water

- 2 cups brown rice, uncooked

- 1 can no-salt black beans

- 3 cloves garlic, minced

Instructions:

1. Bring the water and rice to boil, simmer for 40 minutes.

2. In a pan, cook the black beans with their liquid and the garlic for 5 minutes.

3. Toss the rice and beans together, and serve.

Nutritional Value Per Serving:

Calories 220

Carbohydrates 45 g

Fats 1.5 g

Protein 7 g

Yucatan Bean & Pumpkin Seed Appetizer

Prep time: 10 minutes

Cook time: 3 minutes

Serves: 8

Ingredients:

- ¼ cup pumpkin seeds

- 1 can white beans

- 1 tomato, chopped

- 1/3 cup onion, chopped

- 1/3 cup cilantro, chopped

- 4 Tbsp lime juice

- Salt, pepper, to taste

Instructions:

1. Toast the pumpkin seeds for 3 minutes to lightly brown. Let cool, and then chop in a food processor.

2. Mix in the remaining ingredients. Season with salt and pepper, and serve.

Nutritional Value Per Serving:

Calories 12 g; Fats 2 g; Carbohydrates 12 g; Protein 5 g

Butter Bean Hummus

Prep time: 5 minutes

Cook time: 0 minutes

Serves: 4

Ingredients:

- 1 can butter beans, drained, rinsed

- 2 garlic cloves, minced

- ½ lemon, juiced

- 1 Tbsp olive oil

- 4 sprigs of parsley, minced

- Sea salt, to taste

Instructions:

1. Blend all ingredients in a food processor into a creamy mixture.

2. Serve as a dip for bread, crackers, or any types of vegetables.

Nutritional Value Per Serving:

Calories 150

Carbohydrates 23 g

Fats 4 g

Protein 8 g

Greek-style Gigante Beans

Prep time: 8 hours 5 minutes

Cook time: 10 hours

Serves: 10

Ingredients:

- 12 ounces gigante beans

- 1 can tomatoes with juice, chopped

- 2 stalks celery, diced

- 1 onion, diced

- 4 garlic cloves, minced

- Salt, to taste

Instructions:

1. Soak beans in water for 8 hours.

2. Combine drained beans with the remaining ingredients. Stir, and pour water to cover.

3. Cook for 10 hours on low. Season with salt, and serve.

Nutritional Value Per Serving:

Calories 63; Carbohydrates 13 g; Fats 2 g; Protein 4 g

Brown Rice & Red Beans & Coconut Milk

Prep time: 10 minutes

Cook time: 1 hour

Serves: 6

Ingredients:

- 2 cups brown rice, uncooked
- 4 cups water
- 1 Tbsp olive oil
- 1 onion, diced
- 3 cloves garlic, minced
- 2 cans red beans
- 1 can coconut milk

Instructions:

1. Bring brown rice in water to a boil, then simmer for 30 minutes.

2. Sauté onion in olive oil. Add garlic and cook until golden.

3. Mix the onions and garlic, beans, and coconut milk into the rice. Simmer for 15 minutes.

4. Serve hot.

Nutritional Value Per Serving:

Calories 280; Carbohydrates 49 g; Fats 3 g; Protein 8 g

Black-Eyed Peas with Herns

Prep time: 10 minutes

Cook time: 1 hour

Serves: 8

Ingredients:

- 2 cans no-sodium black-eyed beans
- ½ cup extra-virgin olive oil
- 1 cup parsley, chopped
- 4 green onions, sliced
- 2 carrots, grated
- 2 Tbsp tomato paste
- 2 cups water
- Salt, pepper, to taste

Instructions:

1. Drain the beans, reserve the liquid.

2. Sauté beans, parsley, onions, and carrots in oil for 3 minutes.

3. Add remaining ingredients, 2 cups reserved beans liquid, and water.

4. Cook for 30 minutes.

5. Season with salt, pepper and serve.

Nutritional Value Per Serving:

Calories 230

Carbohydrates 23 g

Fats 15 g

Protein 11 g

Chapter 8: Plant-Based Snacks for Morning and Afternoon

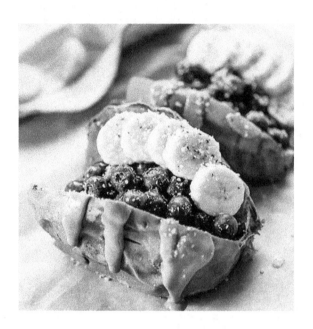

Commended Foods and Dishes

You can eat snacks such as the following:

- Roasted chickpeas

- Avocado lassi

- Apples

- Chia mushroom

- Macaroons

- Chocolate chip cookies

- Fudge

Foods to Avoid

- Dark Chocolate

- Roasted Peanuts

- French Fries

- Candy

Examples and Recipes of Well-Balanced Plant-Based Snacks

Strawberry Mango Shave Ice

Prep time: 5 hours 30 minutes

Cook time: 0 minutes

Serves: 3

Ingredients:

- ½ cup superfine sugar, divided
- 1½ cups mango juice
- 1 diced mango
- 32 oz diced strawberries
- ½ cup coconut, toasted

Instructions:

1. Add one cup of water and sugar to a pot over high heat and boil.
2. Remove from heat and add two more cups of water.
3. Freeze this mixture stirring once in 40 minutes.
4. Take a blender and add all remaining ingredients and blend until smooth.
5. Strain into a container with a pouring spout.
6. For serving, add ice into glasses and pour juice and mixture over them.
7. Serve and enjoy.

Nutritional Value Per Serving:

Calories 366 ; Fat 5.5 g; Carbohydrates 82.4 g; Protein 2.7 g

Chocolate Avocado Mousse

Prep time: 10 minutes

Cook time: 10 minutes

Serves: 6

Ingredients:

- 1¼ cups almond milk, unsweetened

- 1 lb. dark chocolate, chopped

- 4 ripe avocados, peeled and chopped

- ¼ cup syrup of agave

- 1 tbsp orange zest, finely grated

- 2 tbsp puffed quinoa

- 2 tsp sea salt

- 2 tsp pepper flakes

- 1 tbsp olive oil

Instructions:

1. Heat almond milk in a saucepan. After 5 to 10 minutes, add in chopped chocolate.

2. Take all remaining ingredients and blend them till they become smooth.

3. Mix both and let cool for a while.

4. Refrigerate for about 2 hours before serving.

Nutritional Value Per Serving:

Calories 540

Fat 43.5 g

Carbohydrates 61.2 g

Protein 6.1 g

Fudge

Prep time: 10 minutes

Cook time: 5 minutes

Serves: 18

Ingredients:

- 1 cup vegan chocolate chips

- ½ cup soy milk

Instructions:

1. Line an 8-inch portion skillet with wax paper. Set aside. Clear some space in your refrigerator for this dish as you will need it later.

2. Melt chocolate chips in a double boiler or add chocolate and almond spread to a medium, microwave-safe bowl. Melt it in the microwave in 20-second increments until chocolate melts. In between each 20-second burst, stir the chocolate until it is smooth.

3. Empty the melted chocolate mixture into the lined skillet. Tap the sides of the skillet to make sure the mixture spreads into an even layer. Alternatively, use a spoon to make swirls on top.

4. Move skillet to the refrigerator until it is firm. Remove the skillet from the refrigerator and cut fudge into 18 squares.

Nutritional Value Per Serving:

Calories 21; Fats 1.2 g; Carbohydrates 2.2 g; Protein 0.2 g

Chocolate Chip Cookies

Prep time: 20 minutes

Cook time: 0 minutes

Serves: 20

Ingredients:

- 1½ cups roasted, salted cashews

- 8 oz pitted Medjool dates

- 3 tbsp coconut oil

- 2 tsp vanilla extract

- 2 cups old-fashioned oats

- 1 cup semi-sweet or dark chocolate chips

Instructions:

1. Line a baking sheet with parchment paper.

2. In the bowl of a food processor, add the cashews, dates, coconut oil, vanilla, and oats.

168

3. Pulse until combined, and all lumps are broken up.

4. On the off chance that the batter appears to be dry, add 1 more tbsp of coconut oil and a sprinkle of water. Mix in the chocolate chips.

5. Divide the mixture into 18 to 20 tbsp-size balls and place them on the prepared baking sheet. Using the palm of your hand, delicately press down each ball into flat circles. Move the sheet to the refrigerator for 10 to 15 minutes or until cookies are firm.

6. Serve and enjoy.

Nutritional Value Per Serving:

Calories 207

Fat 9.4 g

Carbohydrates 28.1 g

Protein 4.2 g

Peanut Butter Ice Cream

Prep time: 20 minutes

Cook time: 8 hours

Serves: 20

Ingredients:

- 1 cup dark chocolate chips

- 3 cans coconut cream, divided

- ¼ cup peanut butter

- ½ cup granulated sugar

- 2 tsp vanilla extract

- ¼ tsp salt

- ¼ cup graham cracker crumbs

Instructions:

1. Reserve ½ cup of the coconut cream and add the rest to the blender along with peanut butter, sugar, vanilla extract, and salt.

2. Blend until smooth and freeze the mixture for 2 hours.

3. Heat the remaining ½ cup of the coconut cream in a small pot over low heat until it starts to boil.

4. Remove the pot from the heat and add the chocolate chips to the coconut cream.

5. Let this sit for 5 minutes then stir the mixture to combine the chocolate and the cream. The chocolate chips should be completely softened by this point.

6. Let the mixture cool to room temperature.

7. Meanwhile, take out the frozen mixture and mix with the coconut cream chocolate mixture and graham cracker crumbs in a bowl.

8. Let cool for 8 hours in the refrigerator.

9. Scoop out and serve chilled.

Nutritional Value Per Serving:

Calories 154

Fat 11.9 g

Carbohydrates 12.5 g

Protein 2.1 g

Cinnamon Apples

Prep time: 20 minutes

Cook time: 1 hour

Serves: 4

Ingredients:

- 2 apples
- 1 tsp cinnamon

Instructions:

1. Pre-heat stove to 220°F.

2. Core the apples or cut them into rounds with a sharp blade or mandolin slicer.

3. Place them in a bowl and sprinkle them with cinnamon. Use your hands to make sure the apples are coated completely.

4. Arrange the apple cuts in a single layer on a silicone tray or a baking sheet lined with parchment paper.

5. Bake for 1 hour then flip the apples.

6. Bake for 1 more hour. Then, turn the oven off and leave the sheet in the stove until it cooled down.

7. Serve when desired or store in a sealed container for up to a week.

Nutritional Value Per Serving:

Calories 33; Fat 0.1 g; Carbohydrates 9.1 g; Protein 0.2 g

Roasted Chickpeas

Prep time: 10 minutes

Cook time: 25 minutes

Serves: 4

Ingredients:

- 1 can chickpeas, rinsed, drained
- 2 tsp freshly squeezed lemon juice
- 2 tsp tamari
- ½ tsp fresh rosemary, chopped
- 1/8 tsp sea salt
- 1/8 tsp pure maple syrup or agave nectar

Instructions:

1. Preheat stove to 400°F. Line a baking sheet with parchment paper.

2. Toss all ingredients together and spread the chickpeas out on the baking sheet.

3. Roast for around 25 minutes, stirring the chickpeas every 5 minutes or so. Note, until the tamari and lemon juice dry up, the chickpeas will seem delicate, not crunchy.

4. Serve warm or at room temperature for a snack.

Nutritional Value Per Serving:

Calories 290; Fat 10.2 g; Carbohydrates 40.3 g; Protein 10.9 g

Baked Sesame Fries

Prep time: 10 minutes

Cook time: 20 minutes

Serves: 4

Ingredients:

- 1 lb. Yukon potatoes, gold, cut into wedges, unpeeled
- 1 tbsp avocado, grapeseed
- 2 tbsp, seeds, sesame
- 1 tbsp potato starch
- 1 tbsp, yeast nutritional
- Generous pinch salt
- Black pepper

Instructions:

1. Preheat stove to 425°F.

2. Delicately oil a baking sheet of metal or line it with parchment paper.

3. Toss potatoes with all of the ingredients until covered, if seeds don't stick, drizzle a little more oil.

4. Spread potatoes in an even layer onto the prepared sheet and bake for 20 to 25 minutes, tossing once halfway through, until the potatoes become crispy.

5. Serve with desired toppings.

Nutritional Value Per Serving:

Calories 192

Fat 5.9 g

Carbohydrates 32.6 g

Protein 2.8 g

No-Bake Coconut Chia Macaroons

Prep time: 2 hours

Cook time: 0 minutes

Serves: 6

Ingredients:

- 1 cup Shredded Coconut

- 2 tbsp Chia Seeds

- ½ cup Coconut Cream

- ½ cup Erythritol

Instructions:

1. Combine all ingredients in a bowl. Mix until well combined.

2. Chill the mixture for about half an hour.

3. Once set, scoop the mixture into serving portions and roll into balls.

4. Return to the chiller for another hour.

Nutritional Value Per Serving:

Calories 129

Carbohydrates 5 g

Fats 12 g

Protein 2 g

Avocado Lassi

Prep time: 5 minutes

Serves: 3

Ingredients:

- 1 Avocado
- 1 cup Coconut Milk
- 2 cups Ice Cubes
- 2 tbsp Erythritol
- ½ tsp Powdered Cardamom
- 1 tbsp Vanilla Extract

Instructions:

1. Combine all ingredients in a bowl. Mix until well combined.
2. Press the mixture into a rectangular silicone mold and freeze for an hour to set.
3. Slice for serving.

Nutritional Value Per Serving:

Calories 305

Carbohydrates 9 g

Fats 29 g

Protein 3 g

Vegan Fudge Revel Bars

Prep time: 1 hour

Serves: 12

Ingredients:

- 1 cup Almond Flour
- ¾ cup Erythritol
- ¾ cup Peanut Butter
- 1 tbsp Vanilla extract
- ½ cup Sugar-Free Chocolate Chips
- 2 tbsp Margarine

Instructions:

1. Mix together almond butter, coconut flour, erythritol, and vanilla extract in a bowl until well combined.

2. Press the mixture into a rectangular silicone mold and freeze for an hour to set.

3. Melt the chocolate chips with the margarine for 1-2 minutes in the microwave.

4. Pour melted chocolate on top of the mold and chill for another hour to set.

5. Slice for serving.

Nutritional Value Per Serving:

Calories 160; Carbohydrates 5 g; Fats 14 g; Protein 5 g

Chapter 9: Non-Plant-Based Foods

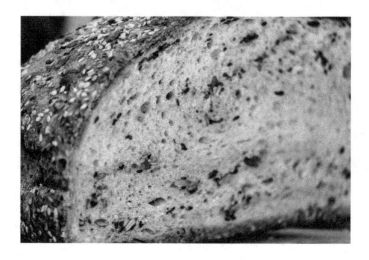

Dairy Free Cheese

Although some soy-, nut-, and rice-based "cheeses" are marked as "non-dairy," they include some form of casein or whey protein. To be safe, buy products labeled "vegan," and read all the ingredients thoroughly, paying attention to words like rennet, evaporated milk powder, or casein. You can also make your own dairy-free cheeses from cashews.

Bread

This fact may be a disappointment for plant-based eaters. The truth is that many famous national brands add non-plant-based ingredients to their bread, like milk products. To find completely plant-based bread, look for one that is made only from whole grains and contains active cultures or other added ingredients like nuts, seeds, or even legumes.

Granola

Granola is usually made with raw grains, dried fruits, nuts, and seeds that are mixed with a sweetener and either butter or oil. The best solution is to prepare the granola yourself.

Non-Dairy Creamer

These creamers can include milk products, such as sodium caseinate, a milk protein. Look for vegan-friendly creamers instead.

Soup Stock

Using bouillon or stock from a carton or can while making soup at home may be very convenient, but many vegetarian stocks or even "mock" chicken stocks may contain a small amount of animal fat or other animal products. To be safe, make your stocks from leftover veggie scraps, seaweed, or herbs sprinkled in water, or look for packages that say "no animal-derived ingredients."

Orange Juice

Orange juice contains omega-3 fatty acids that can have traces of fish oil. Margarine, olive oil, and bread may contain fish-based rather than plant-based sources of omega-3 fatty acids. While on a plant-based diet, don't drink boxed juices. Make fresh-pressed juices, or buy juices that are 100 percent juice and don't contain any additives.

Veggie Burger or Sausages

Many brands add a small amount of milk or eggs to their products. To avoid animal products, choose foods that are made from organic soy (and not isolated soy protein, which is harmful), whole grains, tempeh, or nuts and seeds, with just veggies and herbs added. Or make your own veggie burgers and sausages.

Pasta

Eggs are a main component of pasta. Buy only dried pasta—it's only made of whole grains and water. While eating out, make sure that pasta you are going to eat is egg-free.

Chapter 10: Tips for Flavoring Your Plant-Based Foods

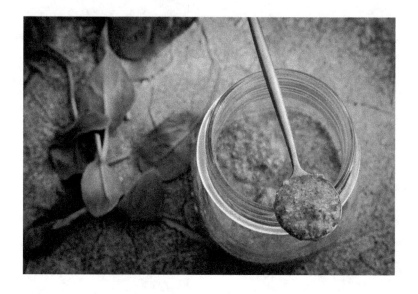

You can flavor your plant-based foods as shown below:

Basil Pesto

Tomatoes, Balsamic Vinegar, Mint, Fruit, Garlic, Eggplant

Spicy Cilantro Pesto

Almonds, Olive oil, Cilantro leaves, Fresh lemon juice, Red pepper flakes, Black pepper.

Spicy Red Pepper Sauce

Garlic, Ancho chilis, Lemon, Garlic, Olive oil

Tomato Sauce

Thyme, Oregano, Red pepper flakes, Basil

Salsa Verde

Tomatillo powder, Ground chiles, Lime peel, Powdered honey, Onions, Garlic,

Chapter 11: Plant-Based Diet Meal Plan

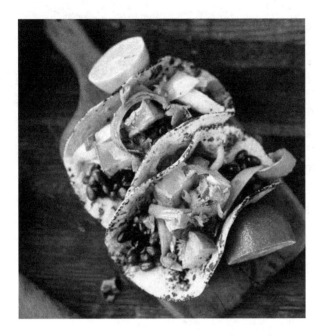

Are you ready to boost the nutrition, flavor, and energy you get from your food? It can all happen at once! I put together these meal plans to show you how to make delicious plant-based meals that give you balanced nutrition and nourishment to fuel your day.

Day 1

Lunch – Cashew Siam Salad

Dinner – Summer Harvest Pizza

187

Day 2

Lunch – Avocado and Cauliflower Hummus

Dinner – Whole Wheat Pizza with Summer produce

Day 3

Lunch – Raw zoodles with avocado 'N Nuts

Dinner – Spicy Chickpeas

Day 4

Lunch – Cauliflower Sushi

Dinner – Farro with Pistachios & herbs

Day 5

Lunch – Spinach and Mashed Tofu Salad

Dinner – Millet and Teff with Squash & Onions

Day 6

Lunch – Cucumber Edamame Salad

Dinner – Brown Rice Tabbouleh

Day 7

Lunch – Artichoke White Bean Sandwich Spread

Dinner – Healthy Hoppin' John

Day 8

Lunch – Buffalo Chickpea Wraps

Dinner – Beans & Greens Bowl

Day 9

Lunch – Coconut Veggie Wraps

Dinner – Black Beans and Brown Rice

Day 10

Lunch – Cucumber Avocado Sandwich

Dinner – Yucatan Bean & Pumpkin Seed Appetizer

Day 11

Lunch – Lentil Sandwich Spread

Dinner – Butter Bean Hummus

Day 12

Lunch – Mediterranean Tortilla Pinwheels

Dinner – Greek-style Gigante Beans

Day 13

Lunch – Rice and Bean Burritos

Dinner – Spicy Chickpeas

Day 14

Lunch – Ricotta Basil Pinwheels

Dinner – Summer Harvest Pizza

Day 15

Lunch – Delicious Sloppy Joes with no Meat

Dinner – Beans & Greens Bowl

Day 16

Lunch – Spicy Hummus and Apple Wrap

Dinner – Brown Rice Tabbouleh

190

Day 17

Lunch – Sun-Dried Tomato Spread

Dinner – Butter Bean Hummus

Day 18

Lunch – Sweet Potato Sandwich Spread

Dinner – Brown Rice & Red Beans & Coconut Milk

Day 19

Lunch – Zucchini Sandwich with Balsamic Dressing

Dinner – Black-Eyed Peas with Herns

Breakfast, Snack, Lunch, Afternoon Snack, Dinner, Evening Snack

Morning: Homemade granola

Snack: Avocado lassi

Lunch: Buffalo chickpea wraps

Snack: Roasted Chickpeas

Dinner: <u>Black-eyed Peas with herns</u>

Snack: <u>Cinnamon apples</u>

FAQs About Plant-based Diet

Going plant-based diet is a new thing in the world today. However, there are many unanswered questions that people have about eating plant foods. The lack of information about these foods is what makes people skeptical about changing their diets. This chapter will take a look at the common questions people have concerning plant-based diets. Answers to these questions will be provided to help you stay informed about these foods and why you need to transition today.

Is Going plant-based diet Difficult?

The mere fact that you will only be eating plant foods doesn't mean that it is difficult to switch to veganism. Honestly, it is easy to switch. You only need to decide to change and commit yourself to the process. The most important thing would be to develop a habit where you eat the recommended foods from your diet plan.

What Is the Best Plant-Based Meat Alternatives?

Switching to plant foods means that you will have to replace your meat with plant-based sources of protein. There has been a huge concern

192

about whether plants can offer adequate protein nutrients that are typically obtained from animal products. Well, there are plenty of plant options that offer this nutrient, so you shouldn't be worried. Ideal meat alternatives include tempeh, seitan, soya, and jackfruit. Instead of choosing chicken, you should choose tempeh. If you love deli meats, seitan would be a preferable replacement.

Is It Okay to Combine the Keto Diet with Veganism?

If you are trying to lose weight, then there is a good chance that you have heard of the keto diet option. Basically, this is a low-carb, high-fat diet. The diet aims to transform your body into a fat-burning machine by ensuring that it is constantly in a state of ketosis. Having said this, it is almost impossible to bring the two diet options together. The keto diet depends on eating a wide array of foods for the weight loss strategy to work. Consequently, some of the foods you will be required to eat include cheese, meat, and yogurt. As a vegan, these are some of the foods you need to avoid. So, a keto diet will not work when sticking to plant foods.

What Are the Recommended Supplements When Eating Plant-Based Foods?

Following concerns that plant-based foods might not be adequate in providing the body with certain nutrients, it is recommended that you should take supplements. Well, depending on what your body needs, your choice of the supplement will vary. Therefore, before buying any supplement, it is usually advisable to consult with your physician. Common supplements that you should consider taking include vitamin B12, omega-3 fatty acids, and vitamin D.

How Can I Start a Plant-Based Diet?

The best way of transitioning to a new, plant-only diet is by taking small steps from the get-go. Break down your monthly goals into weekly goals. The change doesn't have to be immediate for it to be effective. The first few weeks should see you switch from eating meat to replacing your meals with meat alternatives. Gradually, you should try new recipes to keep things exciting. While doing this, you should make sure that your set goals are realistic. Don't forget the importance of educating yourself about the new direction that you are taking. This guarantees that you understand why plant-based diets are good for your body.

What If I Am Not Ready to Go plant-based diet?

Of course, there are instances where you are not ready to change completely. However, this should not discourage you from realizing that you will still benefit from increasing the quantity of vegetables on your plate. Going vegan is more than just the diet. You will have to switch to an entirely new lifestyle where you develop and nurture a compassionate attitude towards animals. Before switching completely, why don't you try being a vegetarian first and see how it goes?

Can I Get All the Nutrients I Need from Plant-Based Foods?

Yes. You can get all nutrients from eating plant foods. Filling your plate with a wide array of vegetables will help ensure that your plate is full of proteins, vitamins, carbohydrates, and other important minerals. Nonetheless, there are particular nutrients which you should be mindful of, like protein, calcium, and vitamin B12, among others. Studies have shown that getting these nutrients from plants is not easy. Therefore, to free yourself from the worry of missing these nutrients on your plate, it is advisable to use supplements.

Are Plant-Based Foods Budget-Friendly?

Plant-based foods are affordable. A common misconception people have is that plant-based foods cost a lot. This is not always the case and it shouldn't deter you from eating healthy foods. There are a few tricks you can use that can help you cut down the cost of buying these foods. For instance, buying your groceries in bulk is a great way of making sure that you don't have to visit the store more than once a week. Additionally, buying locally and seasonally will help you find the best deals in the market. Hunting for discounted deals in the store is another reliable way of saving money when shopping for plant foods.

Is It Still Okay to Eat Pizza?

With the popularity of plant-based lifestyles today, most foods have their meatless versions. This means that you can eat a plant-based diet pizza without worrying about whether animals have been mistreated for you to enjoy your meal. Chefs have revolutionized the idea of creating vegan food versions to ensure that dieters can still enjoy their favorite delicacies.

Do Plant-Based Diets Help with Weight Loss?

Yes. Eating plant-based foods can give you a huge boost to your weight loss campaign. Nevertheless, you should not set your mind towards losing weight alone. This will drain a lot of energy from you if things fail to work out as expected. Instead, pay attention to improve your general health by eating plant-based dishes. This way, you will develop a positive attitude concerning your health improvement efforts. Ultimately, you will lose weight naturally and enjoy a healthy lifestyle where you don't have to feel as though you are sacrificing tasty foods in order to shed some pounds.

Are Vegetarians and Vegans Healthier and Happier in the Long Run?

Definitely yes. Scientifically, plant eaters tend to live longer than people who eat animal products. First, you should understand that plant foods will reduce the risk of diseases such as diabetes and cancer. Moreover, these plant foods are of great importance to your heart's health. Hence, you will enjoy a healthier life free from diseases that might hinder you from enjoying your existence on earth.

Where Do plant-based dieters Get Protein?

Dieters will often worry about getting adequate proteins from plants. Surprisingly, plants can provide one with the recommended daily protein intake. Ideal plant sources of protein include chickpeas, almonds, lentils, tempeh, tofu, quinoa, and peanuts. Ensuring that your body gets enough protein is vital as the nutrient will help you feel satiated. Additionally, it promotes weight loss and muscle strength.

Are Plant-Based Diets Rich in Fats?

Most people are stuck in the perception that fats can only be obtained from eating dairy products and other meat products. Sure, these foods are rich in fats, but it should be noted that they are rich in unhealthy fats that usually lead to health complications. Plant foods, on the other hand, are a rich source of unsaturated fats. Therefore, plant foods are the best sources of healthy fats since they will not cause any negative health effects by eating them.

Are Plant-Based Diets Safe for Children?

Yes, it is safe for a child to eat plant-based foods. However, this should be done by following a plant-based diet plan that puts emphasis on getting all the nutrients that the body needs. Remember, for a child, animal products such as fish, eggs, and dairy products could be included in their meals. This warrants that you don't have to turn to supplements to ensure that certain nutrient requirements are met. More importantly, as a parent, you should take up the responsibility of educating yourself on ideal ways of meeting the recommended intake of vital nutrients such as calcium, iron, vitamin D, vitamin B12, and several others. Consulting with a physician before letting your children try the diet is key to making sure that you don't pose a risk to their health.

Is It Necessary to Get Rid of All Animal Products from My Diet?

Yes. If you decide to start the plant-based diet lifestyle, you must stop consuming all animal products including milk and honey.

Will Eating Plant Foods Help Boost My Athletic Performance?

Contrary to what many people believe, eating plant foods can lead to better athletic performance. The fact that your diet lacks meat doesn't mean that you will not develop your muscles. There are thousands of athletes who maintain their high performance while eating plant-based foods. Your athletic performance depends on the nutrients you take in. Consequently, you should strive to fill your plate with a balanced diet of plant foods.

Conclusion

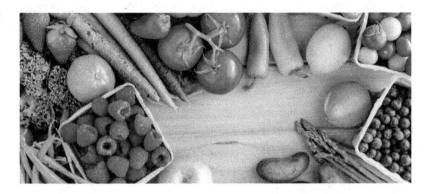

There is a growing concern for healthy living as more and more people are facing difficulty in maintaining healthy lifestyles. Unfortunately, we no longer know what is good for our health. This is because the world today is corrupted with too much unfounded information. Scientific theories have been formulated around our health and this is what makes things confusing. As we look for options for curing diseases, we find ourselves settling for remedies that often do more harm than good. Truly, this is a dilemma that most people face. Sometimes you are convinced that a particular solution will work for you, only to realize later that it is leading to other health complications.

Surprisingly, we all know that our health is dependent on what we choose to eat. Despite this knowledge, we are still not disciplined enough to eat the right foods. Often, we resort to eating junk and engaging in sedentary lifestyles. We know that this is what leads to cancer, diabetes, heart disease, and other terminal and chronic illnesses. So, it beats understanding that we indulge in eating habits that harm us. Following what has been said in this manual, you have a solid understanding of eating plant-based diets. This is one of the best ways to be kind to your body.

A plant-based diet is a diet that is comprised of minimally-processed vegetables, fruits, legumes, whole grains, nuts, and seeds. There are varying ways in which one can stick to a plant-based diet. This is what leads to a huge difference between vegetarians and vegans. Many people assume that vegetarians and vegans are the same. However, the dieters vary as they engage in eating plant-based foods in different ways. Vegans are strict with their diet as they do not eat meat and other animal products. Moreover, to them, being vegan is more than just a diet; it is a lifestyle.

Beyond health, our planet will also benefit from our eating plant foods. These foods will lead to lower greenhouse gas emissions. Over the years, going green as a solution to global climate change has not been enough. Therefore, people must embrace plant foods since that choice will safeguard our beautiful environment for future generations to enjoy.

If you are thinking about changing your diet today, you should understand that this is a lifetime decision that will ensure you enjoy a healthy lifestyle. To succeed in your transformation, you should first begin by finding your motivation. Make it clear to yourself why you want to go vegan or become a vegetarian. Knowing your motivation will help you to maintain focus when things get bumpy. Of course, the change may not be that easy because you will have to overcome many temptations. So, it makes sense that you should have a solid reason as to why you should continue eating right.

In addition, your body needs time to change. You can't force it to adapt overnight to a new diet plan. You must go through a smooth transition. The last thing you need is to be discouraged and abandon your new plant-based diet. Therefore, start by choosing a few dishes that you love the most. Try out different recipes to add some excitement to the process. While doing all this, make sure your environment is supportive of the path you are taking. This means that your kitchen should be organized and filled with plant foods only. Storing meat products will only tempt you to stray from your dietary goals. Ditch these products and replace them with plant-based alternatives.

The people around you will also play a huge role in helping you change for the better. If your friends and family are not supportive of the idea, then you will find it more challenging to switch. Sure, these people might not understand why you are changing to a plant-only diet. Thus, you should make a point of educating them about your decision. Help them realize that there are many health benefits of eating these foods. In time, they will see the positive changes in you and could be motivated to follow your path. In line with this, you should take advantage of social media pages and connect with like-minded individuals. Associating with people who have similar health goals will help you maintain your focus and motivation. Moreover, they will encourage you during difficult times. Their real-life experiences will also act as a benchmark to what you expect to witness as you remove animal products from your diet.

Most importantly, you should commit yourself to the process in order for you to reap maximum benefits. Set practical goals and strive to achieve them. If you want to lose weight by eating plant foods, then set clear goals. If you are looking to manage a chronic disease you are suffering from, commit yourself to the cause. With commitment, you will develop a habit easily. This will make a huge difference in following a plant-based diet without feeling that you are sacrificing anything. Look at the bigger picture and understand that you are doing this for all the right reasons. After all, you are what you eat.